COMMON SENSE CANCER

MY SURVIVAL STORY

ANN MARIE FRASER

Common Sense Cancer
My Survival Story

Edited by: Onika Nkrumah-Lakhan

Graphic Artist: Oneil Wright

Medical & Not Healthcare Advice Disclaimer:
The daily program, protocols, best practices, products, services, suggestions, statements, and health information written in this book have not been evaluated by the United States Food and Drug Administration and are not approved to diagnose, treat, cure or prevent disease. They are provided as informational resources only. They are not intended to be an authority on medicine, a substitute for cures for any disease, including cancer in all its forms, a substitute for advice from a healthcare professional, a substitute for medical diagnosis and treatment and should not be considered or relied upon as such. They are not intended to be patient education and does not create any patient-physician relationship. You should consult your physician about interactions between medications you are taking and nutritional supplements mentioned in this book. The author, editor, graphic artist, doctors, companies, website-owners and individual names listed in this book shall not be liable for any illness or adverse effects caused by the use or misuse of information and products presented in this book.

Printed in the United States of America

Common Sense Cancer
My Survival Story

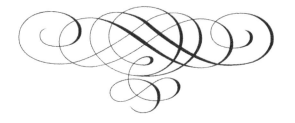

Dedication

This book is dedicated to my husband and best friend, Lenny. You are the hero who stood by me, through it all.

Acknowledgments

My gratitude is extended to several persons without whom this timely and relevant book would not be possible. First, I must thank Jesus Christ, my Lord, and Savior, for His sustaining love, grace, and mercies towards me; my husband Lenny, for his steadfast love and support, my daughters Nyala and Aletea for their constant encouragement to get this book written. Thanks to my Mom, Lucitta, my brother-in-law Ashield, my sisters Ingrid, Lystra, and Erica, for helping with many of my responsibilities during my recovery. I give special thanks to my formers bosses Mr. Trevor H.C. Baker, Mr. Larry J. Bailey, Mr. Seth Bardu and Mr. Ebenezer Agboka for being so kind, in granting me time off while I worked on my health.

Special, special thanks to Mrs. Janet Holmes and Mrs. Gwen Shorter, Lifestyle Educators, who took me into their homes and cared for me like I was their own. They lovingly shared their special natural remedies and protocols that helped nurse me back to health. I thank the following doctors who helped me along my journey: Dr. Millicent Comrie, MD, Dr. Phyllis Hyde, MD, Dr. Rachael Ollivierre, MD and Dr. Mamon Wilson, Gospel Medical Missionary Evangelist.

Let me also thank from the bottom of my heart the following ministers from various congregations, for their continued prayers and counsels even during my current years of remission:

Bishop Carl C. Alexander, Tabernacle of Praise of All Nations.

Bishop Mervin Harding, Grace Deliverance Temple, Church of God.

Pastor Eugene Phipps, Jesus The Good Shepherd, Reformed Episcopal Church.

Pastor Winston Stevenson, Evangelist, NEC of Seventh Day Adventist.

And finally, a very special Doctor from Mexico with the initials S.V, for his brilliance and unique method of helping me and others in successfully fighting cancer.

Contents

Preface

My dear friend, Judy Brown, once said to me, with an effervescent joy in her eyes, "Girl, one day your biggest survival experience, will become a bestselling story. The world really needs this inspiration."

My reply to such a confident statement was: "Thank you. And, I also hope that it positively impacts the lives of every person who reads or listens to it because my story is solely due to God's glory!"

It occurred to me a long time ago that sometimes all it takes to change the world is the testimony of one person, who has been transformed by an experience; far beyond their understanding. This person also knows that all things work for the good of the Lord. That person is ME! I want to be clear that this book is not intended to be an authority on medicine or as a cure for any disease, including cancer in all its forms and should not be considered as such. Neither is this book written to force my religious views and convictions on you. My success story is solely intended to be an inspiration to you, as you traverse life's journey, as you cope with your various life experiences and as you strive for a healthy lifestyle.

I have learned that nothing is more specific than life's uncertainty. Everyone is prone to experience the consequences of life's choices. Admittedly, this can be very frightening to some persons, especially with the inevitable reality that things will happen in our lifetime that is unexpected and will lead us down a difficult path. And, it is worse yet, if this path is called breast cancer.

I am a survivor of this crucible and not only have I overcome it, but I am a better person today.

As the title of this book proclaims, Common-Sense Cancer, I believe that I should apply wisdom in everything I do, even if it is merely using my God-given common-sense. Common-sense, you might ask?

It's interesting that some people are very skeptical about ordinary or common things. These are things that seem too easy or accessible, appear senseless or non-essential, without taking into consideration that 'common' does not mean 'obvious.' Sometimes, we circumnavigate to avoid the very things that are there to help us. And more so, if it has to do with a disease like cancer, more specifically, breast cancer, some people will even choose to live in denial of it.

In this book, you will find a wealth of information on the common-sense methods I followed for dealing with my breast cancer including, resources on spiritual wellness, prevention, guides, and healing methods that were used for my benefit.

The purpose of this book is to help others battling this disease, those living in fear of it; to help the healthy in mind and body to avoid cancer and to motivate and encourage others. These are others whom I would not otherwise be able to meet personally, whether they be rich or poor, famous or unknown of every race. We have lost so many wonderful and promising people to cancer, who might still have been with us, had they only known other things that they could have done.

As an overcomer, I recognize God's grace and mercy throughout my journey, and I strive to expand His claim in my life to reach others. In fact, I take no credit for anything good that has ever happened to me and will ever happen: "I can do all things only through Christ who gives me strength." - Philippians 4:13.

This book will open your understanding of your greatest powers through God. You have a marvelous mind and body that God has given you, and He wishes above all things that you succeed: *"For I know the plans I have for you," declares the LORD, "plans to prosper you and not to harm you, plans to give you hope and a future."(Jeremiah 29:11)*

One secret to success is to begin to feel successful right now. It starts in your mind. Ask God to bless you with success, then believe that it is done. Indulge your mental and physical senses on information found in the word of God, for example; you may start by reading the book of Psalms. Then, watch how God will place people in your life to provide mentorship, self-development, and opportunities for success, as He has done for me. Dear reader, please understand that God will only answer your prayer if you intend to use your success to do good, and to bless others.

In my opinion, many books written on the topics of self-improvement, inspiration, health and wealth attainment have a central message: *you have power through God's Grace.* So, wake up to the fact that you have the power of God behind you. It is time to discover your full potential to maintain a prosperous and healthy lifestyle.

Never limit yourself to what you think you can do, see yourself doing what you want to do. I wanted to survive, bring encouragement to my readers even if I were to suffer re-occurrences. Hopefully, my story will inspire women to make mammograms, breast self-examinations, and healthy lifestyles a priority. This to me is common-sense!

Realize that when the praises go up, the blessings come down. Every good thing that you desire, you can attain. Keep your thoughts and feelings in full alignment with God's will, then be happy, thankful and watch your blessings flow, as the purpose of your life and what you need for your journey of success becomes a reality.

I am greatly honored and thankful for the opportunity to share my unique story, to teach, support and to highlight the giftedness of all medical workers, physicians, lifestyle experts, and Common-Sense practitioners. As you read, I pray that you will be inspired to:

1. Live in awareness of your health.
2. Take responsibility for your actions.
3. Appreciate the love and support given by your significant others. If you feel like you do not have supportive people in your life, "there is a friend that sticketh closer than a brother" (Proverbs 18:24 KJV) Find that friend within your circle. Also, remember that Jesus Christ is not just your Savior but also your Friend.
4. Seek the purpose for your life.
5. Accept that you can do all things through Jesus Christ.

I hope that after reading this book, you will be motivated to make common-sense decisions.

*-**Ann Marie Fraser,** Author.*

Foreword

It is a pleasure to present to you Ann Marie Fraser's book, *Common Sense Cancer: My Survival Story.* For more than twenty years I have known Ann Marie as a brilliant, professional, and humble Christian woman, a loving wife and mother. She has maintained an unshakeable faith and trust in God through all the vicissitudes of her life and in her recent relentless battle against cancer.

It was on Thanksgiving Thursday of November 2007 that an intruding killer struck her body with a violent thrust sending tremors of anguish and fear throughout her being. Subsequent diagnoses confirmed it. She was a victim of cancer!

The story of Ann Marie's survival is chronicled in her fascinating book. Stay with her as she struggles with the treatment modalities from which she must choose: whether the traditional medical procedures or an alternative regiment which skeptical doctors frequently characterize as unscientific and quackery. Give attention to the not so *"common-sense"* strategies she employs in managing her battle.

This book is filled with health principles, spiritual encouragement, and great suggestions to improve your health. It is a "must read" if you are struggling with illness. It will motivate you to press ahead, and never give up on achieving your goals and dreams.

What makes this book useful and different from other inspirational books is Ann Marie's unique common-sense and practical approach to fight the battle you may be facing. She shares with you the steps she took while battling cancer and making her personal story come alive.

I join with Ann Marie in believing that this book will encourage you to have an abiding trust and faith in God because He hears the cries of His children. I am convinced that *Common Sense Cancer: My Survival Story* will inspire you towards a better quality of physical and spiritual health.

Rupert W. Young, D.Min., LCPC
Retired Minister.

Introduction

"What Cancer Cannot Do" Cancer is so limited. It cannot cripple LOVE – It cannot shatter HOPE – It cannot corrode FAITH – It cannot destroy PEACE – It cannot kill FRIENDSHIP – It cannot suppress MEMORIES – It cannot silence COURAGE – It cannot invade the SOUL – It cannot steal eternal LIFE – It cannot conquer the SPIRIT."

- Anonymous

The Root of My Perseverance

Whenever a vicious assailant attacks someone, the common-sense reaction is to fight back to avoid being killed. I was stricken by vicious cancer, but I didn't surrender. I fought back!

I fought back God's way. I survived my cancer attack by utilizing Special Weapons and Tactics (SWAT). My special weapons were: my faith in God, educating myself about breast cancer, working with my medical and naturopathic doctors, using low dose chemotherapy and natural remedies, the love and support of my family and friends, and a positive mindset. I call this a Synergy!

I was born on the beautiful island of Trinidad and Tobago. I grew up with my grandmother and my mother who were self-made, successful businesswomen. They taught me discipline and about the benefits of dedication and hard work. They operated a family grocery and club. My grandmother also sponsored an annual community fair for the children in the neighborhood. From an early age, I learned how to interact with community members, to operate a successful business, and why it's so important to give back to the community.

There is no doubt that my upbringing and sense of community played a significant part in my will to persevere and survive. However, it was not enough to combat that assailant called breast cancer. I would have been thrown down to an early death, had it not been for God's grace and mercy.

My victory was possible because of the direct intervention of a loving God. I am wrapped up in His love.

Love is the bridge between human needs and divine supply. This bridge will never fall. In fact, all it takes to demonstrate the awesome providence of God in your life is to find ways to share your experience. There are lovely, caring people in your life. There are those who will not only fight cancer with you but will also ensure that telling your story becomes a reality.

Love yourself, especially if you are fighting a deadly disease. By loving yourself, you will recognize your motivations and why you may need to make changes, as well as realize your full potential in finding solutions to your problems. The one thing that can hold you together during any terrible ordeal is the love of Jesus. Love yourself fully, because God first loved you. When you love yourself, you develop the power within you to love others.

There are many life lessons learned from my unwelcome experience.

Lessons such as, how to persevere when the odds are stacked up against you, how to appreciate life and not take time for granted, how to be grateful for the special people in your life and very importantly, how to be successful and win!

If you are ready for success, willing to affect change and to embrace God's power and magnificence, then I hope my story blesses you.

Your Creator has imparted infinite power to you. His power is the only source of energy you need.

The idea of success is an inborn quest that many pursue. Whether it is a spiritual, financial, educational, physical or emotional success, it can be attained by merely following the instructions of God.

I found a sense of great joy knowing that God has promised us success when we follow His formula:

"The book of the law shall not depart out of thy mouth; but thou shall meditate therein day and night, that thou mayest observe to do according to all that is written therein: for then thou shalt make thy way prosperous, and then thou shalt have good success."

-(Joshua 1:8 KJV)

I have always tried to maintain a purpose in my life. I am also gradually learning more about how God works, and how He heals and restores. He guides our steps and helps us make lifestyle changes necessary for good health. Sometimes we physically feel like we cannot make those changes; emotionally we feel afraid of getting unfavorable results; financially we might be at our lowest, but we must always remember that God is ever-present. Therefore, He can meet us where we are and restore us to where we need to be.

As humans, we are often tempted to ask, "why me?" Why did I get cancer, even though I was a practicing vegetarian? Why do I struggle to make ends meet even though I'm a Christian? I am living proof that God heals but, I also believe that some of our most potent spiritual breakthroughs come through adversity or illness.

Sometimes the Lord may allow us to suffer and experience disease, poor health, and hardship. The reason for this is that, He can often teach us things through suffering, that we would never be receptive to, during times of comfort and prosperity.

I find it is to make us stronger. Nevertheless, God is merciful, and this book is not about the 'why' of illness but about the 'how' you can be healed!

For your healing to begin to manifest, you must agree on a conscious level to be successfully healed. When you accept, choose a method of healing. The method you employ, whether preventive or curative, primary or secondary or merely a "common-sense" Synergy, may help you to be on your way to a healthier lifestyle.

The word of God is perfect, and it states that God desires for you to have good health and prosperity. You should believe that whatever you ask for, you will receive it. There is no room for doubt.

Medical doctors help their patients by following established medical procedures that include physical examination and testing, which identifies the root of their illness. Then, they try to help patients by prescribing medications, various treatments or surgical procedures that assist in the recovery of the patient.

Medical doctors are scientific, they are trained to understand what they can prove, but battling cancer, for me, required a combination of the physical and the spiritual. I used a common-sense synergistic approach to dealing with my breast cancer.

In the subsequent chapters, I hope you will be encouraged by the steps I took to achieve my recovery.

Here are some tips:

1) When dealing with cancer, you must determine what you want, which is total healing. Don't let your mind tell you that it's not possible to achieve it. Consider doing a synergy. This is a great way to fight cancer. In my experience, the majority of cancer patients rely heavily on just one method of treatment. For instance, they would do chemotherapy, surgery, and radiation only, others are convinced that they can beat cancer by using natural herbs alone; still, others try prayer alone, under the mistaken notion, that prayer without action, will bear results. I chose what seemed like common-sense to me, I considered my options and decided to create a synergy: a combination of all the methods.

2) Share your situation with your significant others. You will need their undying devotion on this journey. If no one else knows, then, how can they help you? Or, even pray for you?

3) Set goals and resolve to achieve them gradually and sequentially. Some will be minor, and some major, for example: changing your eating habits. Remember to

maintain a plan for your success. Be specific about the results you expect. Don't aim only to stop your cancer from spreading, instead, strive to starve and kill it!

4) You must visualize what you expect. By faith, see the tumors and cancer cells disappear forever. Imagine it clearly in vivid detail.

5) Don't be afraid to face this challenge. The Bible states that God has not given us the spirit of fear. Fear does not promote good health. Now is the time to exercise common-sense judgments and soundness of mind. Remember, God is in control.

6) The Creator has already established master techniques for total restoration. One may find many resources on how to meditate on God's Word. But, it takes more than just meditation and medicine to maintain health. It takes a complete lifestyle change. It takes a love that never dies. Like the love of my husband who supported me through the pain and suffering or like the love of my best friend, Marlene Robinson, who always encouraged and wished the best for me.

7) Finally, persevere. Occupy your mind with positive thoughts. Get rid of every flicker of doubt. Know that whatever you think, focus on and work hard at, that is what you are going to get more of. So, let your belief be perfectly secure and settled in God.

PART 1

LIVE IN AWARENESS

OF YOUR HEALTH

Chapter 1

A Rude Introduction

*"You beat cancer by how you live, why you live
and in the manner in which you live."*
- Stuart Scott

Thanksgiving Thursday with an Intruder

I have always led a busy and full life: business, family, church, travel, seminars, meetings, helping others and fun. So, the day that I first discovered something was terribly wrong with my body was the same day I had decided that I was going to be my best no matter what would come my way. But, I was in for a rude introduction to a traumatic experience that neither, I, my husband nor my daughter, who was at home with us, expected nor did we understand.

It was the afternoon of Thanksgiving Thursday, 2007. It was a lovely day. Sweet, stirring gospel music saturated the air, and my mind was occupied with its symphony. The mood was set for something great and I was getting dressed to visit my sister-in-law, Dorothy Richardson.

After all, who wouldn't want to be with the extended family for Thanksgiving? It was always fun to enjoy the songs, games, and dinner that Dorothy and her children would prepare for the whole family each year.

My husband, Lenny and my daughter, Aletea were already dressed. I might have kept them waiting, but our optimism for the evening was quite evident.

As we were about ready to leave home, I felt a very sharp pain, like a needle prick. When I touched my breast, I felt a lump and immediately I knew that something was wrong.

Pain and lump in my breast? The thought was a like a swift intruder that I immediately wanted to chase away. An incredulous, depressive mood overcame me and I began to feel like my legs were made of spaghetti.

The reason why I felt depressed was that I instinctively knew something was wrong and I was too shocked to admit that this was most likely the dreaded signs and symptoms of the big "C" in my body. Then, the shocking reality hit me like a lightning bolt-BREAST CANCER?

My mind was racing, and my chest felt like, somebody wearing steel-tip boots was standing on it. *Could this be what I'm thinking?* And if it is, *how could this happen?* I had been a vegetarian for about twenty-seven years: *Wow! How could this happen?*

I collapsed clumsily into the nearest chair and called out with a voice that fell somewhere between fatigue and sleepiness to my husband and daughter and told them that I wasn't feeling well. They were understandably confused and kept asking me, "What happened?"

I could see the concern in their eyes even in my confusion. But, it was not too long before the answer gradually became obvious to them. Something must be wrong!

I no longer wanted to go to the Thanksgiving dinner, so I stayed at home by myself. I had an opportunity to think about what might be happening.

Waiting in solitude was my choice, in hindsight, it was a bad idea because cancer feeds on stress and negativity, yet at the same time, thinking about the situation was unavoidable. I couldn't ignore it.

After Shock: A Blow from Cancer

As a person who belongs to a large Christian denomination, I have witnessed on many occasions, ministers and other professional speakers being introduced to an audience. I have always noticed that the way a person is presented, has a lot to do with the expectations and interests of their audience.

Life gives us many unwelcome experiences and being introduced to cancer is just one of them.

Throughout the years, I have learned that the real purpose of life is devotion to God, as our Creator, and to live in awareness of our health.

If we are not practicing health principles, then we are choosing to allow our bodies to begin to fail us.

What do you do when you are introduced to something or someone you didn't anticipate? If it's a person's unannounced arrival at your home, you might feel awkward, embarrassed, irritated, surprised, or even angry!

This is exactly what it's like finding out that your body is a host, to the most unwelcome, unexpected guest ever, Cancer! It's the last thing you would have on your expectation list. Now, what are some of the obvious repercussions of such a rude awakening to breast cancer?

Cancer affects your peace of mind. The body feels the burden of mortality and the mind anticipates things beyond rational thinking. You just don't know what might happen. The uncertainty of your future seems unbearable, and you may feel as if you have been given a death sentence and this is a legitimate feeling because so many people are being diagnosed every day.

"In the U.S. for example, about 11 million Americans alive today—one in 30 people–are either currently undergoing treatment for cancer or have done so in the past."[1]

---

[1] Cancer survivor. Taken from paragraph two, sentence three. Retrieved from https://en.wikipedia.org/wiki/Cancer_survivor

Coping and Hoping during Cancer

Just because breast cancer is a rude introduction to something deadly, does not mean that it has to be a death sentence. It does not have to be the end of your journey. Knowing this is crucial to your survival.

Never allow yourself to feel as if there is no hope, always believe that there is something you can do and that you will beat your cancer. Never think that it is too late. To accept defeat is to reject your life's purpose.

These feelings of hopelessness are to be expected but should not be overly entertained. Different people have different ways of coping. This can be through denial or acceptance of the situation. Whichever coping mechanism you accept, one thing is sure. Something is drastically wrong with your body, ignoring it is NOT the answer, it needs to be addressed as soon as possible.

Eviction on Cancer

There is no need to panic when you have a firm foundation of faith. When such unwelcome intrusion takes place, just know that you have the God-given power to evict your unwanted visitor and begin the process of healing.

Simply put, any situation can be solved at the initial stages, if you believe in the power of God to overcome and by this same faith, take decisive action.

Whatever direction you take remain focus on pushing forward. It is safe to say that total healing begins in the mind. If you believe that you will be healed, then you will be in a better frame of mind to look at your options without fear and to overcome.

By now, you might have a clearer picture of my Thanksgiving Thursday's experience.

No Quick Step Away from Cancer

Transitioning from my usual daily activity one moment to registering what I was feeling the next, was no quick step. My thoughts were confused for a while until I snapped my mind back to reality.

That evening when I felt that sharp pain, I just needed solitude, I wanted to be alone to process this sudden, terribly odd discovery of something alien in my body. This is a typical reaction to breast cancer.

This rude introduction to breast cancer on Thanksgiving Thursday initially plunged me into feelings of doubt, fear, and concern. Luckily, these feelings of doom and gloom were later replaced with meaningful common-sense action.

That same evening, I began checking my breast for more lumps. I had hoped they would not be found. But, my hopes were soon chased away by a barbarous discovery.

Chapter 2

The Lump Check

"We must embrace pain and burn it as fuel for our journey."
– Kenji Miyazawa

Off to the Doctor with a Vengeance

The week after Thanksgiving, I got out of bed, read my Bible and prayed about the lump I was feeling. Then, I called and made an appointment to see a breast doctor. Just knowing that the lump was there gave me an uneasy feeling. I felt like my blood pressure had risen, but I was so glad that I had listened to my instincts and took my symptoms seriously.

The doctor immediately suggested a needle biopsy after she had examined the lump. "Well, Mrs. Fraser," she said in a measured tone, "We will have to do a biopsy, to confirm whether the mass is benign or malignant."

Even though I was willing to have the test done, I was nowhere near ready to hear the truth of the results. Understandably, my questions queued up, and the minutest probabilities began to invade my thoughts. *What more would they discover? What was the worst thing that could go wrong? Was I even ready for this?*

We scheduled a checkup for the following week, and soon after, we did the biopsy. Afterward, the doctor called to tell me that it was negative. Great, thank You, Lord! I breathed a sigh of relief, but not for long, because the lump was still painful and annoying. So, off to the doctor, I went again. "Well," she said, "We did a biopsy already, and the results were negative." I insisted that the pain was increasing: "Well, instead of doing another biopsy, let's just do a lumpectomy and take the lump out, and then we will send it to the lab for testing," she said to me.

I sat uneasily and remained silent for a moment, trying to gather my frantic thoughts and suppress my panic. "OK," I said, finally.

I had never done a breast surgery before that. It wasn't something I was eager to do, but I had to do it, like it or not.

I believe one of the keys to my success, has been my ability to be realistic about things. There are some things in life you may not want to do, but you will have to do it anyway.

A common-sense approach means taking deliberate action, at all costs, wishful thinking is never enough.

Do It Anyway; Be Tough on Cancer

I want you to know, that regular checkups, which can detect early signs of breast cancer are vital.

Although breasts self-exams may not show a clear benefit, yet doctors conduct them all the time. I discovered my lump and was later diagnosed signifying the significance of breasts self-checks.

Therefore, "It's important for women to be familiar with how their breasts look, and to check them regularly. This will help them become aware of any changes or abnormalities as they occur."[2]

---

[2] Holland, K. (2016, January 13) What does a breast cancer lump feels like? Learn the symptoms. Medically reviewed by Christina Chun. (2017, October 11) Retrieved from https://www.healthline.com/health/what-does-breast-cancer-feel-like

A Lump Check is A Life Check

A lump check is a life check. This realization fueled my quest for answers. I began to practice the best technique of checking for lumps, in and around my breasts. I did it in the shower, in the mirror and sometimes in bed. I believe this is important for your benefit and peace of mind. Some women are so occupied with the demands of their daily routine, they ignore the essential aspects of their health.

It's important to be aware of your health, this simply means making common-sense prioritization of what matters most to you and your family. I believe that women should know that a lump check done the right way can prevent bright days from giving way to frightening nights of bewilderment and pain. It can avoid the heartache of family members and friends. It could make the difference between dreams fulfilled and dreams unfulfilled.

A simple lump check can save your finances from depletion. A simple lump check can be the wake-up call to new beginnings. This is a common-sense decision for every woman to make. In the next chapter, I will show how I assaulted the creeping killer who intruded upon my peace.

Chapter 3

Symptoms of a Creeping Killer

"Cancer does not have to kill you because you are its host. Keep your immune system strong. It is your internal defense that will help fight cancer for you. Develop that mindset."
-Ann Marie Fraser

The operation went according to plan. The lump was removed and it was sent to the lab. The results indicated that it was a benign tumor. I breathed a sigh of relief: "Thank you, Lord," I whispered. I cannot express in words the joy I felt that day. I was relieved of my anxiety. The female doctor said assuredly, "See! It was nothing to worry about."

The doctor's words were comforting momentarily. Although, why my breast was still experiencing such excruciating pain remained a mystery. It was a mystery that required further investigation.

It Was Always There, That Tricky Cancer!

I had my breast bandaged up after the surgery, but when the bandage came off, I was not at peace. The pain was intermittently so annoying. I had to put my hand on the area, at times, to get ease.

What happened next was terrifying. One day, I felt the spot where the lump was removed. I was shocked, I realized that the lump was back! Whatever it was, it just came right back. So, I called my doctor and made another appointment to see her.

When I returned to her, the doctor examined it and explained: "A lot of African-American women have fibrocystic breasts, so it isn't anything to worry about," she said: "It's just scar tissue from the surgery, don't worry, it will soften and eventually go away."

My dear readers, that's not what happened. What I felt did not go away but gradually continued to grow. Now, my lump was spreading like an octopus's tentacles.

As time went on, the lumps continued to get harder. I could not believe it! What I was experiencing in my body did not coincide with the doctor's explanations. This feeling of uncertainty was not helpful for my situation. Not only was I now dealing with the symptoms of a creeping killer in my body, but also, I found myself doubting a doctor who was either unaware of the cancer's presence or was just too busy to follow up with me. In my opinion, she wasn't overly concerned.

A Time to Respond

The symptoms of cancer increased my understanding that every woman must take responsibility for her health. When things are not going the way you expect it to, own it, and fix it.

I was not satisfied with the doctor's response, knowing how my breasts felt, only kindled more questions in my mind. Something was just not right about the whole situation. I needed greater assurance. Common-sense to me meant seeking a second opinion.

In the quest for a second opinion I visited and counseled with my regular Gynecologist. When she realized that I was still feeling pain she agreed that I needed a second opinion and she recommended a new breast doctor.

I visited that new doctor, who ran some more tests and redid my biopsy. I recall the day as the doctor dogged deeper into my flesh. I remember screaming because it was so painful.

This time, the results confirmed my worst fears, now my continuous pain made more sense. "Mrs. Fraser, I'm sorry. I wish the news were better. You have breast cancer," she said, in a regretful tone.

When the doctor confirmed I had cancer, I could not believe her. Her lips were moving, but her words could not register. I refused to hear anything after the initial bad news. My first thought was my husband and my children. How would I tell them? My family and friends! My job! My clients! My whole life seemed to flash before my eyes.

Just imagine, it was not too long ago when the first biopsy and the lumpectomy of my breast tumor came back benign. Now, I was hearing that it was malignant and in an advanced stage! I never considered the possibility that cancer could develop so swiftly in my body.

Pain on the Train

The train ride from Manhattan to Brooklyn, that day, was one that I will never forget. I had just been given a cancer diagnosis, and some would even say I was given a death sentence. I sat on that train, absorbed in my world. It felt like I was swimming around in a fish tank, the outside sounds of the world were muffled, the sights blurred. I tried to block out everybody around me and whatever loud, annoying conversations they were having. All I could think about was what I had just been told. As I got off the train, I had already decided to accept my diagnosis and start calling on the Lord Jesus Christ for guidance.

Let me assure you that when you sincerely call on Him, He listens.

I Hate Cancer!

Having cancer spread through your body is one of the worst feelings to bear. I have felt the pains of childbirth, experienced headaches and cramps, but none compared to the alarming feeling of having a creeping killer inside of you.

If someone asked me: "How does it feel to have had, breast cancer?" I probably would find it difficult to give a quick answer. I am cognizant of the fact that the details of how cancer spreads and how it feels can be quite uncomfortable for some individuals, especially when they are young and looking forward to a cancer-free future.

According to the National Cancer Institute (NCI) dictionary of cancer terms, metastasis is:

"The spread of cancer cells from the place where they first formed to another part of the body. In metastasis, cancer cells break away from the original (primary) tumor, travel through the blood or lymph system, and form a new tumor in other organs or tissues of the body. The new, metastatic tumor is the same type of cancer as the primary tumor. For example, if breast cancer spreads to the lung, the cancer cells in the lung are breast cancer cells, not lung cancer cells."[3]

"Cancer can spread in 3 ways:

- Invasion – the tumor grows into surrounding tissues or structures.
- Through the bloodstream – cancer cells break away from the tumor, enter the bloodstream and travel to a new location in the body.
- Through the lymphatic system – cancer cells break away from the tumor and travel through the lymph vessels and lymph nodes to other parts of the body."[4]

"If the cancer spreads beyond the breast and the nearby lymph nodes, it's considered advanced, or metastatic. The most common places breast cancer spreads to, are the lymph nodes, liver, lungs, bones, and brain."[5]

I have done many imaging tests, so that my doctors saw what was happening inside my body and whether the disease had spread. How cancer spreads is one

---

[3] NCI Dictionary of Cancer Terms. Metastasis. Retrieved from www.cancer.gov/publications/dictionaries/cancer-terms/def/metastasis
[4] Cancer-something you cannot be prepared for? (2017, August 5) Category: Medicine. Retrieved from https://mypassionmedicine.wordpress.com/category/medicine/
[5] Reviewed by Pathak, N. (2018, January 30). Retrieved from www.webmd.com/breast-cancer/when-breast-cancer-spreads

thing, but, one must also deal with the pain of cancer.

"Pain is an indicator of something being wrong with the usual cause being an injury or an illness. In either case, the nervous system notifies the brain of a problem by sending a pain signal through the nerves. When the signal is received, the pain is felt.

Every kind of pain is transmitted in the same manner, including pain due to cancer. As not every type of cancer causes similar pain, the type of pain you feel can give an indication about a broad cancer type at least. For instance:

Deep and aching pain is usually caused by a tumor that is present close to the bones or that grows into the bones. This kind of pain caused by cancer is mostly bone pain.

Burning pain is caused by tumors that press on parts of nerves. Cancer treatments like surgery, radiation and chemotherapy can sometimes damage nerves and give rise to a burning feeling.

Phantom pain is the sensation of pain in an area where a body part, like a breast or an arm, has been removed. The pain is felt even though there is no body part because of the nerve endings in the region continue to send the pain signals to the brain."[6]

---

[6] What does cancer feel like? Pain: Obvious Symptom That Cancer Can Cause. Retrieved from https://www.newhealthadvisor.com/What-Does-Cancer-Feel-Like.html

What Breast Cancer Feels Like

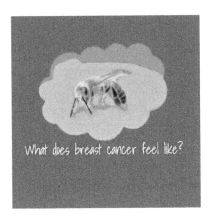

What does breast cancer feel like?

Cancer is a slow killer, and it comes with pain, whether mild or chronic, but no one should be afraid of it. So, to answer the original question, it felt like a bee had stung me. The pain of that sting was so sudden and sharp that I would bawl out. The burning pain continued to move around in my chest, it felt like pins and needles deep in my flesh. Then it would stop, until the next sting. It was an annoying feeling.

Chapter 4

A Choice of Reaction

"You gain strength, courage and confidence by every experience in which you really stop to look fear in the face. You must do the thing which you think you cannot do" – Eleanor Roosevelt

Don't Panic! It's Only Cancer!

What do you do when you are caught between a rock and a hard place? Or, in my case, what do you do when you are faced with making a life or death decision about cancer treatment?

Should I go the conventional way? I was concerned about weakening my immune system. I was worried about the terrible side effects of the drugs. I thought about losing my hair and my breasts.

Or, should I go totally natural? My health insurance would not cover natural protocols. I would personally be responsible for the entire cost of treatment. There were so many decisions to be made and so little time.

I was conflicted. I could not make a decisive choice, regarding my treatment plan of action. I chose to continue believing that Christ, my Lord, would sustain me.

Every time I felt like panicking, I stopped and refused to give in to cancer. I put all my energy into learning what it took to stay alive, and as healthy as I could.

I could have chosen to ignore the reality at hand. I could have unrealistically wished it would go away like magic! But, I knew that sooner or later the cancer would have to be dealt with. And, the sooner, the better.

Insurance and Assurance: At War with Cancer

Insurance companies may not readily insure individuals who they think are a potential liability. In other words, these are persons whom they figure have a higher probability of death, like cancer patients. Someone like me! As a licensed Insurance Agent, this field is a big part of my expertise, but companies denied me life insurance because of my ill-health. Therefore, I encourage every individual to secure your financial future while you are healthy.

After finding out my diagnosis, the question was: What am I going to do now? I found myself pondering many problems. I'm also a Certified Public Accountant. I do taxes for many clients, and furthermore, this was January, how was I going to get all their tax returns done, having just been diagnosed with cancer? My clients were so loyal that I just did not know how to tell them to go elsewhere. I had so many concerns.

I was thinking about everything I deemed necessary while going through the pain. I had to get through the tax season, and then I would take care of me. This was not good common-sense because the cancer was spreading while I was delaying my decision, but that's what I tried to do.

Usually, the tax season ends on April 15th, however; I did not make it beyond the first week of April. I could not lift my right hand. I could not even lift a pocketbook!

The tumor was bigger in the right breast and cancer had already spread in both breasts and my lymph nodes. Moreover, the pain was so excruciating that at that point I knew that I had to stop working. It was necessary to start figuring out what I had to do to fight my cancer.

Thou Shalt Not!

The breast doctor who diagnosed me did her due diligence in research, and she talked to me in detail. She then expertly and judiciously recommended an Oncologist whom she believed was going to be right for me.

I met with the Oncologist as recommended. He sat with me and laid out my treatment plan. My treatment plan required me to: take two types of chemotherapy in heavy doses, once a week for six months. Then, I would do a double mastectomy to completely remove both breasts, after which I would do heavy doses of radiation.

After hearing the course of treatment, doubt and fear began to creep in. I tried to ask intelligent questions about the treatment plan, which even under the circumstances, I felt was extreme.

"What about trying other natural things?" I asked nervously.

The Oncologist looked at me and said: "Listen, if you don't follow this plan, one day, you are going to just lie down on your bed, and you are not going to be able to get up,"

Then, after reading my questioning face, he added: "You will not be able to move and won't be able to get out of your bed. I will give you six months, and you'll be gone from here."

The Oncologist meant that I would be dead in six months if I didn't follow his instructions! Then, he cautioned me some more: "There will be no discussion about natural or other remedies. Your type of breast cancer is rare. This is serious, okay," he said, with a tone of finality.

"Okay," was my immediate response, although my facial expression betrayed my inner feeling. No patient ever wants to come to their doctor and risk offending them, and we rely entirely on their medical expertise, it can even feel awkward asking specific pertinent questions.

Interestingly, I felt that the good doctor was just doing what he knew best, but when I left his office I knew I was not returning! You will be surprised by what happened, later on in my story.

Regardless of what man can do through medicine, I know personally that God is the one that has the final say. To be clear, I am not advocating that one should not adhere to the prescribed methods of their doctor. I am just telling my truth, about how miraculous God worked in guiding my direction and decisions.

Just like the Biblical character, Naaman, who was told by the prophet Elisha to dip into a murky river seven times before he could be cured of his leprosy. I have learned that when God says seven, six will never be accepted. As humans, we incline to be doubtful, like Thomas (John 20:25), and not trust all the way with our faith.

> "Except I shall see in his hands the print of the nails, and put my finger into the print of the nails, and thrust my hand into his side, I will not believe."

This is what we should understand, never make the Creator your last resort. I know it's not as simple as it sounds, but how can you prove God to work miracles for you, if all you do is try to figure everything out logically? This was it. I had to act, but I didn't necessarily have to do it the 'logical' way. So, what did I do next?

A Natural Approach to Cancer Treatment

The first thing I did was visit Lifestyle Educator, Janet Holmes. Janet Holmes is an amazing woman, having studied to become a medical missionary, she knew the wonderful results that I would experience using natural protocols. As she cleansed my body thoroughly, nourishing my immune system using natural herbs and remedies, I depended on Christ Jesus for ultimate positive results.

It is a once in a lifetime experience to meet individuals like Janet Holmes and Gwen Shorter, who have dedicated their lives to doing God's work and helping people. It was amazing the way how Janet Holmes from upstate New York and Gwen and the late

Rick Shorter, whose Lifestyle Center, I stayed at in Yorba Linda, California, dealt with me.

It does not matter a sick person's background or position in life. Whether they are black or white or whatever nationality they represent. For these amazing human beings, it's about love, and love transcends everything. They understood that God is no respecter of any group or individual. I stayed in both their homes. I learned lots of natural protocols which I will share later in this book. I left with my body feeling cleansed and nourished. My confidence in the Divine was elevated.

Successful People and the Gift of Life:
Lessons learned from Cancer

Successful people cherish the gift of life. The greatest gift that a person has is their good health. A healthy body led by a healthy mind is your greatest asset. This is a huge part of your success. Even if you have millions of dollars, you can't enjoy it, if you are sick. On the other hand, having health can eventually navigate your path to having wealth.

Some people eventually die from the despair of coming to grips with the fact that they have cancer. They become so terrified, that they can do absolutely nothing. They hide it, refuse to talk to others about it, or share their feelings. In my opinion, successful people handle things differently.

Regarding health, successful people know how to react to situations. They learn from the strength of others. When sickness or disability befalls them, they rise above their circumstances and refuse to accept their position as final. A successful person's mindset is never to lay down and die.

When diagnosed with cancer, the only thing to do is to go through it. You can't avoid it. We all want to be strong when faced with life's challenges, but sometimes that strength is hard to access. I tried to be strong for my daughters' sake. Internal weakness is one of the worse emotions a person can face. I worked hard to rise to the occasion and maintain a positive mindset. Honestly, I don't think my children can ever say they saw hopelessness in me.

Dear readers, I hope that I can encourage you not to panic or feel overwhelmed by the many life and death choices that may face you. It's helpful to talk to someone about it, and it is therapeutic to vent your frustrations rather than keep them bottled. Maybe you can begin by communicating with the most significant person in your life, or your doctor, or your pastor. Just know that someone is there for you. Therefore, stop worrying!

Worry Ends Where Faith Begins!

Every person who aspires to maintain a healthy balance would know that there is no benefit in worrying about life's ills. In the Holy Bible, Jesus made this profound statement:

"Therefore, I say unto you, take no thought for your life, what ye shall eat, or what ye shall drink; nor yet for your body, what ye shall put on…" (Matthew 6:25 KJV)

Faith is boldly going with Jesus where you have never gone before and where you would never even dare to go on your own. The Bible describes faith as believing.

"Now, Faith is the substance of things hoped for, the evidence of things not seen." (Hebrews 11:1).

Our Heavenly Dad is Wealthy

There are millions of people who are curious to know if God approves of poverty or riches among humanity.

In the book, *Rich Dad Poor Dad* by Robert Kiyosaki, the author evaluated both his dads. While one is poor, the other is rich. Kiyosaki explained the life lessons he learned from both. However, Dads are human beings, and humans have limitations. God, on the other hand, has no such limits! Your heavenly Dad is wealthy enough to take care of your cancer bill.

I had to exercise my faith like never before. I had to trust in God and believe in His guidance. My heavenly Dad opened doors for me. Without exercising faith that God would take care of the bills, I would not have had the confidence or the resources necessary to fight my cancer.

Drop useless goals:
Take up a weapon against cancer

Remember why you're alive. What do you want to accomplish in life? Know that you need to focus only on the things that will contribute to your recovery and survival. Everything else is wait! Don't make the initial mistake I made, of delaying action until the end of the tax season. I wanted to meet my obligations to my clients, but that was not too smart. Guess what, God forbid, if any one of us were to drop dead tomorrow, life would continue uninterrupted. Your company would hire someone else, and your clients would take their business elsewhere! Direct your energies to the worthy pursuit of good health and the real substance of life.

You may have to drop some things. When you are diagnosed with cancer you can't do everything as before. Figure out which goals are critical for you to accomplish and leave the rest to others. Plan and hope for the future, but don't leave it there; it's time to fight cancer now! You can't slow the world down, so if you are doing too much, slow yourself down. If you are downtrodden and cancer has you frozen in your tracks, then you need to be re-energized with a renewed sense of hope in God

Set aside a particular time for prayer. Time spent in prayer is invaluable. It is our greatest weapon! Adopt a new hobby. Something that will keep your mind active, yet rested and stress-free. A good example is reading books that will keep your thoughts positive and inspired. I started reading the book: 'Desire of Ages' by Ellen G. White. The Lord one day said to His disciples:

"Come ye yourselves apart into a desert place, and rest awhile. Christ is full of tenderness and compassion for all in His service. He would show His disciples that God does not require sacrifice, but mercy. They had been putting their whole souls into labor for the people, and this was exhausting their physical and mental strength. It was their duty to rest."[7]

---

[7] White, E.G, (1990) Desire of Ages. Silver Springs: Review & Herald and Pacific Press, p. 203

Believe that things will be okay. Remember the Great Physician, is working behind the scenes on your behalf.

Chapter 5

Much to Do About Something or Nothing

"The worst thing you can do with any life-threatening disease is sit around all day waiting for the next test. If I die tomorrow, I think I could look at myself in the mirror and say I tried everything I could to live as healthy a life as possible. I did not just sit around and hope that the next treatment might work."

~ Arthur Fowled, prostate cancer survivor

Camping Against Cancer

I learned a lot about my body and how breast cancer was affecting me. The knowledge I acquired helped me make common-sense decisions.

The transition, from my lifestyle pre-diagnosis, to working on my recovery, post-diagnosis, entailed a complete paradigm shift. But, it dramatically increased my odds of survival. I realized that I had to cleanse my system, then begin rebuilding my body. Taking full responsibility for my health, was one of the keys to my survival.

When I went to stay at Janet Holmes' home, I learned a lot about healthy living. I followed almost the same protocols every day while I was there. Here is a daily outline of the ten-day detox and cleansing which I underwent, as the first step in my fight against cancer:

My Daily Program

5:30 AM	Prayer/Devotion/Thanksgiving for a brand-new day of life.
6:00 AM	Ionized Alkaline Water/Lemon
6:30: AM	Mineral Citrus Flush- I Drank 64 ounces in 45 Minutes
8:00: AM	Skin Brushing/Hot & Cold Shower
8:30 AM	Breakfast/Vitamin Shot
10:00 AM	Breathing practice/ Exercise time
11:00 AM	Detox & Fiber Drink/ Ionized Alkaline Water
11:05 AM	Sunlight
11:30 AM	Green Juice/Coffee-Enema
12:30 PM	Rebounder/Infra-Red-Sauna Hot & Cold Shower
2:00 PM	Vitamin Shot/ Ionized Alkaline Water/Rest
3:00 PM	Lunch-Green Juice/Vegetables

5:00 PM	Green-Smoothie/Coffee-Enema /Shower
6:00 PM	Dinner/Green Salad
7:00-9:00 PM	Health-Education/ Ionized Alkaline Water/ Detox Fiber Drink
9:00 PM	Rest/Lights out/Bed

Janet and I began each day with prayer and devotion. As a customary practice, we read Bible verses, praised God and gave thanks for new mercies.

This was followed by drinking ionized alkaline water and doing a mineral flush. The mineral flush had a 'yucky' taste but, all things considered, it was good. Following Janet's instructions, I would sip 64 ounces in forty-five minutes. It flushed out my system real good.

Breakfast was certainly different. Everything was 'live' food. Keep in mind that cancer thrives on dead, cooked foods. Therefore, it is common-sense to eat live food, as much as possible. Breakfast consisted of fruits, usually two kiwis, one tangerine or a couple slices of grapefruit, about fifteen blueberries, sprinkled with a few hazelnuts.

I love fruits. As a vegetarian, I was accustomed to eating plenty of fruits but, one could imagine my dismay, when I realized that there would be no more white bread, no peanut butter, no jelly, no cheese, no fried plantain, no eggs! I was only given fruits and raw 'live' foods! Gradually, I grew accustomed, and Janet's presentation of breakfast on my plate made up for all that I thought was missing.

After breakfast, it was green juices and green smoothies which Janet would blend for me. The green stuff was very good, and I would drink a glass of green juice for lunch daily.

I would consume six ounces of green juice, 2-3 times per day. The combinations were: Barley life green powder juice, kale and apple, sometimes with green algae, red cabbage juice with apple, collard greens with green apple, dandelion with apple, which helps to flush the liver and kidneys, E3 live green juice, which builds up vitamin B12 and helps support T-cells.

I had three ounces of vitamin shots, twice per day, between breakfast and lunch. This is a strong antioxidant drink. The vitamin shot was made up of 1 ounce of Noni, 1 ounce of Acai berry, 1 ounce of Mangosteen fruit and 1 ounce of goji berry. These were all 100% organic juices.

Dinner was usually, a delicious salad with raw, cruciferous vegetables comprised of: baby or spring green lettuce, grated radish, raw chopped broccoli cauliflower, garlic, scallions, tomatoes, avocado, cabbage, collard greens, tofu, and lots of beans.

Regarding the protocols I had to do, I did my best.

It was challenging at times, but to achieve success over cancer, I was willing to remain disciplined. With so much to accomplish in life, some things are difficult, but certainly not impossible.

Laughter is the Best Medicine

There was something else of equal importance that I came to acknowledge while staying with Janet Holmes. Laughter is the best medicine!

Not everyone who wants to help others to recover from cancer will consider it important enough, to talk about the valuable benefits of joy and laughter, despite the situation. But, I intend on sharing with you the benefits I received and hope it will be helpful to you as well.

Throughout my stay at the Holmes' place, there was an audio-Bible being read softly in the background. There was always an atmosphere of calm and a spirit of peace. The memory verse that Janet would recite daily is in the book of Proverbs:

"A merry heart doeth good, like a medicine: but a broken spirit drieth the bones" (Proverbs 17:22 KJV).

Did you know that laughter is such good medicine that it helps relieve and fight stress, headaches, infections, and hypertension? Health Practitioners tell us that laughing produces physical benefits just like those, we get from vigorous, physical exercise. Laughter decreases stress hormones and increases our immune cells and infection-fighting antibodies which, in turn, boosts our immunity to diseases. Laughter also causes the release of the body's own 'natural high' chemicals called, Endorphins.

When you throw your head back and laugh out loud, you are doing yourself a great favor because you are exercising the muscles in your abdomen, chest, and shoulders in your body, it is called a good 'belly laugh' in my native Trinidad. God created laughter because He knew it is good for our health.

Get Rid of Toxic Thoughts and People

I was often tempted to complain and to feel bitter, but I did not allow negative feelings to overcome me. Instead, I learned to endure and exercise self-control. I aimed to remain optimistic. The emotional effect of cancer may systematically cause negative vibes, ongoing feelings of stress, frustration, loneliness, pain, and anxiety. There is also the stigma attached to any terminal illness and, of course, insensitive people who may make thoughtless, discouraging remarks or give pitying looks. Filtering out those toxic thoughts and people is super-important. Some people believe that because you have cancer, you are done, but many survivors will tell you differently, there is life after cancer!

Replace negativity with the positivity of the Almighty. This joy is an experience you receive from being in His presence, it increases your faith, hope, confidence, and encourages you, regardless of your circumstances.

What Should I do?

Life is a combination of probabilities and assurances. Sometimes, it is not that simple, to make the right choices about our health. *Should I do this or should I do that?* Often, the answer is a combination of the available options presented.

What do you do when you are confused or when you have the toughest decision of your life to make on a grave matter? In my case, an Oncologist told me: "Listen, if you don't follow this plan, …I will give you six months, and you'll be gone from here." His solution was to immediately start using chemotherapy, with no time to waste. A regimen of chemotherapy, surgery, and radiation were apparently, my 'only' options. What was I to do when common-sense told me this might not be the best choice, should I risk, going down the unbeaten path or take the established road?

I was unsure about my next move. If I went the natural way, would I have to wait for a long time before I saw results? On the other hand, should I take those powerful drugs and risk destroying my immune system? Medical doctors were saying chemotherapy and radiation while the lifestyle educators were saying: No chemotherapy! No radiation! No surgery!

I was indeed confused. I knew I had to do something because the pain was increasing and I could feel cancer eating at me with the fury of a thousand hungry leeches. Who should I listen to? The fact remained that, I respected both the medical doctors and the lifestyle educators, but my life was on the line, and I had to make the call.

Then, I recalled the lyrics of a powerful song by gospel singer, Tramaine Hawkins called:

'What Should I Do?'
"What shall I do?
What step should I take?
What move should I make?
Oh Lord, what shall I do?

I'm going to wait
For, an answer from You
I have nothing to lose
Oh Lord, I'm going to wait
I know You'll come through
With a blessing for me
Please Lord set my soul free
Oh Lord, I know you'll come through

I can't live without Your help
I am weak all by myself
Lord please give me the strength I need
So I can possess eternal peace

Choir repeats

No one else can calm my fears
God alone can wipe away my tears
Glory to the mighty king
In Jesus Christ I have everything

Oh there's no one like Jesus
Who can heal broken hearts
And put them back together again

What shall I do
What step should I take
What move should I make
Oh, Lord What shall I do

I'm going to wait
I know you'll come through" [8]

Prayer: The Answer to My Cancer!

I realized that I had to learn to listen to the voice of God. So, I did what I knew best, I prayed. My husband and I went into fervent prayer. We called on the name of our loving Savior, Jesus Christ. We believed with all our hearts that if, Jesus could give sight to the blind, cause the lame to walk, feed thousands with five loaves of bread and two fishes, turn water into wine, cast out demons, walk on water and raise the dead from the grave, then; we knew He could cancel this deadly cancer from my body.

So, we prayed a prayer of faith and God helped

---

[8] Hawkins, T. Lyrics. What Should I Do?

us to make the right decision. It was not long after that God opened the door of opportunity. The phone rang. It was my dear friends, Gwen and Rick Shorter, calling to introduce me to J.P., a Registered Nurse. J.P. was a woman with an incredible story, and her experience provided a rapid response to our prayers.

J. P.'s Story

"When J.P. was diagnosed with Non-Hodgkin's Lymphoma, a cancer of the lymph system, in 1980, the disease was extensive. It had branched out throughout her body, to her pelvis and abdomen. She was told that this was an incurable form of cancer. She was treated in Houston, Texas for four years.

At the end of this period, J.P.'s doctor told her, that the institution had nothing more to offer her, she was sent home without a further appointment. She had suffered bone marrow depression from all the radiation she had been given and was told that this damage would be permanent.

A Barley Grass Miracle

Shortly, thereafter, J.P. learned about barley grass, a fine green powder. Barley grass is a 'live' food, full of vitamins and minerals, which delivers enzymes whole to your body, unlike the fractionated, incomplete synthetic supplements, which ironically, can create bodily imbalances, because the body is unable to effectively process them.

Feeling battered, bruised and broken from the long years of ineffective treatments, J.P. began taking barley green, without any expectation that it would do her any good at all. However, four months later her tumors had disappeared! Her blood tests showed that her bone marrow was functioning normally again and subsequent biopsies showed healthy bone marrow.

This was J.P.'s introduction to the world of whole food concentrates. Despite her medical background, she did not understand before now, that when cells were fed these concentrated nutrients and when all their nutritional needs were met, healing and restoration could begin from the inside out. Her immune system started to improve with the much-needed nutrients. Her largest tumor, under her left arm, began to soften and quickly dissolved. It was a barley grass miracle!

After being in remission for eighteen years, J.P. slowly began to relapse. The cancer had returned with a vengeance. J.P. felt that it was likely that she would die of the lymphoma that she had been fighting for so long. She had continued to take large amounts of barley green, eating raw foods and drinking fresh-squeezed vegetable juices every day. She even went to a health institute, where for three weeks she ate all raw foods, went on juice cleanses and even squeezed wheatgrass juice, which she not only drank; but gave herself rectal installations of its green juice.

J.P. even made poultices with the juice, which she applied to her tumors, but to no avail. When she went to see her Oncologist again, he really had nothing to offer her, his first comment to her was: "J.P., your neck is ugly!" The large tumors in her neck caused her to have a heavy, distorted look. She also had a large mass in her right pelvis, which pressed on nerves that caused pain when she walked.

J.P. knew about some of the cancer clinics in Tijuana, Mexico, but she didn't have confidence in any of them. A couple of doctor friends suggested a clinic in the Dominican Republic, after checking that out, she decided to go there. Before she and her husband could leave they found out that the same organization had recently opened a clinic in Tijuana. So, J.P. chose to go there, instead.

After three weeks of treatment, it became evident that her cancer was growing rapidly, leaving her to wonder, if the treatment, itself, was accelerating her disease!

One day, she had a sonogram of her neck. Right there on the screen, in living color and gory detail, she could see, the tremendous blood supply to the tumors. Now, it made sense why they were growing so rapidly. Then, to her shock and horror, she saw a tumor pressing on her carotid artery, the large artery that supplies the brain with blood! This tumor was not yet impeding blood flow, but that was going to happen very soon. She also knew that when this happened, she could go blind, become a vegetable or die, to name a few of the nasty possibilities.

One day, she and her husband, ate lunch in Tijuana for the first time. They went to a small health food restaurant. While there, a gentleman came in, ate and when he was about to leave, he spoke to the couple. It turned out that he was a doctor at another clinic, and when he found out that she had lymphoma, he immediately told her of the good success rate, his clinic had in treating this type of cancer. J.P. took his business card, but she and her husband had no intention of changing clinics.

A mere six days later, she felt the tumor pressing on her carotid artery. The artery had now started to block blood flow. That night, she packed her neck with ice, to relieve any swelling. J.P. then told her husband good-bye. By then, she had done her grieving, she felt ready for whatever was next. Her relationship with the

Lord was strong and she was ready to go to sleep, until the resurrection day! Her husband told her, that if she made it through the night, they would try the new clinic, the doctor in the restaurant, had told them about. Fortunately, she did make it through the night and by eleven o'clock, the next morning, she was being seen by Dr. S. V. *(The author was unable to reach Dr. S.V, for permission to use his name in this book)*

The doctor, that they had met in the restaurant worked for Dr. S.V.

J.P. had been against taking chemotherapy or any toxic drugs. However, she was so far gone, by the time she went to this clinic, in a last-ditch effort to save her life, that she felt they couldn't do anything more to hurt her.

Within just four days of treatment at Dr. S.V.'s clinic, J.P.'s tumors were no longer visible, and she was no longer under any immediate threat. J.P. believes that meeting that doctor in the restaurant was a direct answer to her prayers. It was a divine appointment, and she thanks God, every day for His divine timing in guiding her to Dr. S.V!"[9]

---

[9] Pauley, J. (Adapted from the J.P. Story)

A Timely Motivation

I was very much moved, and motivated by J.P.'s story. I decided to use a combination of treatments, a synergy which included, heavy doses of common-sense. At that moment, I believed God was inspiring me. If I were in the first stage of cancer, then I would try only natural remedies and no drugs. I believe that natural remedies come directly from God:

"The leaves of the tree were for the healing of the nations" – (Rev 22:2 KJV)

Herbs and plants are obviously amazing and their benefits are incredibly effective. But with natural remedies, you may have to allow more time to see results, because of the years of damage done to the body.

Dear reader, my cancer was an aggressive carcinoma which had already metastasized. My own common-sense told me that I had to fight it more aggressively. God's plan is the natural way, and I understood that the natural way might take longer to work.

J.P.'s story was motivational for me. After sharing her amazing testimony with Lenny and me, we knew without any doubt, that God had answered our prayer.

A Synergistic Approach To Cancer, Worked for Me!

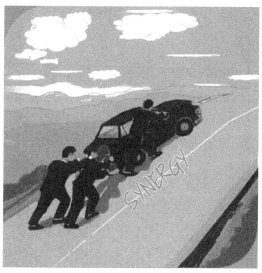

"A synergy is the interaction of two or more forces so that their combined effect is greater than the sum of their individual effects." [10]

For example, if I had to push a car up a hill by myself, it would be quite a challenge. However, if I have the combined strength of three men helping me, the collective effect would most likely get the job done.

I was running out of time, and my cancer was spreading. This was the 'common-sense' behind my decision to use a combination of both treatments. I

---

[10] Leveillee, C. About Synervation. (A). Retrieved from http://www.synervationpt.com/about.html

decided to do the conventional chemotherapy, radiation, and surgery, but differently, from how it is usually done in the U.S. I did chemotherapy and radiation in very low doses.

I underwent a double subcutaneous mastectomy, instead of removing both breasts completely, which is what is done with a double mastectomy. In a subcutaneous surgery, they cut under the skin, and remove just the cancer cells and breast tissues.

I believe in a synergy approach. No one method alone may work. I know people who fought cancer using only the convention treatments and others who tried only the natural remedies. I even know some people who were in denial and paralyzed by inaction. In all those scenarios, sadly someone lost their battle, so I chose to use a synergistic approach instead. I am not a doctor, and I cannot recommend what you should do. I do believe however, that going to any extreme can be dangerous. Therefore, exercise good judgment and 'common-sense.'

PART 2

TAKE RESPONSIBILITY

FOR YOUR SITUATION

Chapter 6

Inner Calm

"It's about focusing on the fight and not the fright."
~Robin Roberts

Hurricane Cancer: You Have Power over Cancer

Battling cancer is like going through a storm. You will experience waves of nausea and winds of despair, then, an uneasy calm before another storm of feeling anxious, vulnerable and out of control. Sometimes you feel like your life is suddenly out of your hands. It is at these times that you should lean on the people you trust. Realize that you cannot fight this alone.

It is essential to exercise your power of choice and find ways to regain control. I was fortunate, not only, to live through my cancer storm, but also literally, one of the worse hurricanes that passed through the Virgin Islands, hurricane Irma! I saw, firsthand, the devastation and destruction of a paradise island. Then, I saw that after a storm dies down, there is calm. Therefore, concentrate on getting through your storm. Get through it. Relax, because the calm will come.

Relax!

Being diagnosed with cancer is by far one of the worse things that can happen to anyone. I decided that I was going to take my worse experience and turn it into my best recovery. I wanted to live to win this battle. I asked God to guide me and give me the strength to do what it took to survive. Through it all, I learned to relax.

I found out during my research that:

"currently nearly 65% of adults diagnosed with cancer in the developed world are expected to live at least five years after the cancer is discovered."[11]

I didn't realize until much later, what a gift God had given me, during the cancerous stages. My gift is peace of mind.

If your situation is terrible, whether it be cancer, or a divorce, or the loss of a child, and you are

---

[11] Cancer Survivor. Quote found in paragraph two, sentence two. Retrieved from
https://en.wikipedia.org/wiki/Cancer_survivor

experiencing feelings of despair, hold on, a breakthrough is coming. I want to encourage you, just like the many survivors who had inspired me. Their testimonies lifted my spirit when I felt my worst.

Allow God to Direct and Lead

There is an inner calm that comes over me when I allow God to direct and lead. The Bible says that:

"A man's heart deviseth his way: but the Lord directeth his steps" (Prov. 16:9).

I relied on His direction, grace, and mercy. I firmly believe that God could use my experience to motivate others and to accomplish His will in their lives.

A Cushion of Mercy

God is merciful. He was indeed gracious to me. I often recalled saying to my children: "God is good and you cannot go wrong if you choose to serve Him." Everything in life is a test, but God does not give us more than we can bear, He always provided me a way out as He promised:

"God is faithful, who will not suffer you to be tempted above that ye are able; but will with the temptation also make a way to escape, that ye may be able to bear it." (1 Corinthians 10:13).

I remember someone asking me: "How did this happen to you and you are a vegetarian?" I felt sad at the time, but I knew it was not asked with ill intent. However, I have a different perspective on things. I believe, the fact that I was a practicing vegetarian, was one of the reasons why my immune cells were able to mount a defense and help pull me through, I may not have been so lucky if I were not.

When a person is diagnosed with a severe illness like cancer, they already feel like death is staring them in the face. The last thing they want is for others to make them feel foolish, ashamed, or guilty.

I came to understand I was never promised a pain-free life; life could be brief, and I am not indispensable; that sometimes bad things also happen to good people. Therefore, after I overcame, I endeavored to be even more patient, kind and empathetic to those going through tough situations.

God would always make a way, where it seems like there is none. That is the love of the great God I serve.

Chapter 7

Priorities:
A Matter of Money or the Thorn in My Flesh

"My cancer scare changed my life. I'm grateful for every new, healthy day I have. It has helped me prioritize my life."

-Olivia Newton-John-

Invest in health

It is incumbent upon me to tell you, dear reader, that if you are diagnosed, it does not necessarily mean that you will die. So many survivors prove my point, including me.

As soon as you are diagnosed, however, you

should immediately begin to do the right things to turn your health around.

Since my cancer was aggressive, I decided that my mindset also needed to be aggressive. There were so many expenses that I did not think about before. However, I knew that regardless of how much money I needed, God would come through for me.

When you have been through an experience with breast cancer, fighting hard is the most logical thing to do. At this point, I could not worry about holding on to what was left in my savings account. Either, I was going to use all of my savings on paying for natural remedies and protocols or allow my cancer to grow. Common-sense told me to use every 'red' cent that I had to take care of myself. I figured, once I got well again, I would be able to earn it back.

Nobody wants to have money worries while dealing with a life-threatening illness or to have to choose between spending money and getting better. Common-sense told me that since my breast tumor was in a small part of my body, I should not be overly afraid to fight it. I had to spend a little fortune on my treatments, the type of water I drank, and on natural remedies.

Cancer may be a death sentence, but it does not need to be carried out! Invest in yourself, because you are worth it.

Dealing with Added Insecurities

So, you or someone you know is diagnosed with cancer, and you are confused and frightened. The medical doctors are recommending a treatment plan for you, and the naturopathic doctors are doing the same, family and friends are calling to share things you can try. People are trying to sell you things that are supposedly good for you; a lot is going through your head right now, you are not sure what to do. Believe me, I know, I have been there!

There's a good chance you have lots of questions. You may be struggling with fears about what could happen, concerns about what to tell people, or wondering if you're going to be able to manage your study or work. You might be worried about what the hospital would be like or how your family would cope. Additionally, you're probably feeling a whole range of emotions, some of which can be overwhelming.

There was never a time when I thought I would lose the fight against cancer. Even when I was skin and bones, my weight had dropped to 110 pounds, also when my veins darkened from the chemotherapy, even when I lost breast tissue and lymph nodes, and even when a doctor told me that I might not make it! I kept on fighting. My mind was resolute. I wasn't about to wait for the curtain to close on my life. I was convinced that only God had the final word.

Beating cancer begins in the mind. Ask God for healing and believe He will answer affirmatively. I prayed and did not doubt. I also, understood that Faith without works is dead. I had to change my eating habits and lifestyle. I had to be obedient to the will of God, and when He healed me, it would be for His glory. This is one reason why I wrote this book!

Talking to people who have been through cancer, or care for others with cancer can make you knowledgeable of what to expect. It lessens your concerns, keeps you optimistic, and make you feel more in control. It also makes you more confident about making those financial decisions, as you hope for a future without cancer.

Give even during cancer

I recall a fascinating story in the Bible. It was about a poor woman who gave her last penny to demonstrate her love for the Lord. God was impressed with her selfless giving and encouraged others to do likewise.

Although God does not need our money, He will still challenge our faithfulness. We will be tested to give consistently, systematically, and cheerfully. We must not allow fear to limit our giving and constrict our blessings.

I needed all my finances for treatment, but I chose to remain faithful in tithing and giving. When you don't know where the next cent is going to come from, that's the time to be faithful.

Change Your Concept of Ownership

I understand and accept that God owns everything. You may not agree with this perspective, but consider this, no one can take their riches to the grave, and our heirs can quickly lose their inheritance in any number of ways. As humans, we are His custodians or stewards. I asked myself: *Should this be about money? Or the thorn in my flesh which in my case was breast cancer?* I concluded that I should concentrate on getting better, and let God worry about the money.

Since God owns everything, He can give us what we need. He is responsible for our success. We, therefore, have no reason to be fearful in our giving. We are to take responsibility and make beneficial use of what He has entrusted to us. Adolphe Monod said,

"There's no portion of money that is our money and the rest God's. It's all His, He made it all, gives it all, and He has simply trusted it to us for His service..."[12]

---

[12]Monod. A. Quotes. Swiss Clergyman (1800-1856). Retrieved from

The Next Move

My next move against cancer was even more strategic than before. After I went to the Holmes' place for two weeks, and I accomplished so much, I was now ready to seek further help. I was on the threshold of a miracle.

http://www.winwisdom.com/quotes/author/adolphe-monod.aspx

Chapter 8

Once Upon a Time in Mexico

"Do not follow where the path may lead. Go instead where there is no path and leave a trail."
~Muriel Strode

The Last Place on My Mind

The last disease I expected to develop was breast cancer. Similarly, the last place I imagined going for treatment of any disease was Mexico. Going to Mexico was another milestone on my journey to recovery.

My doctor in Mexico was the same physician who had worked with J.P., previously mentioned in chapter five. Our initial contact with him was by phone. I explained my condition and the treatment plan that had been laid out for me in the United States. I was surprised that he spent more than an hour interviewing me, answering my questions and describing how his low dose chemotherapy and radiation method of treating cancer worked.

After listening to him, many of my concerns were resolved. Dr. S.V. explained that I would not have to undergo the heavy doses of chemotherapy, the radiation would be in small measures and I may not have to endure a complete double mastectomy. I felt reassured that I made the right decision to work with this doctor.

Immediately after concluding our interview, my husband and I made plans to travel to Mexico, to meet with the doctor. A few days later, shortly after midnight, we touched down in San Diego, California. From there we traveled to Tijuana, Mexico.

At 9:00 am the next morning, a driver collected us and we were taken to the doctor's clinic which was minutes away from our hotel. When we arrived, we were introduced to four other cancer patients who were also beginning their treatments.

Initially, I was thoroughly examined. They did blood work, bone and pet CT scans, X-rays, and heart EKG tests. All these tests were necessary to assess my current situation with cancer and to develop an action plan.

The following day I began the low dose chemotherapy treatments. After my first dose of only a few units, I realized how critical it was that I did not agree to receive the full dose, as had been outlined for me in the United States.

Before taking the chemotherapy, my blood results reported my white blood cells (WBC) at 8.5. This was very good since normal WBC is between 5 and10. However, by the next morning when my blood was re-tested, my WBC was so low (2.8) that the doctor made a decision not to give me anymore chemo, for the next twenty-four hours.

That same day, I decided to walk back to the hotel which was a couple of blocks away. To my surprise, I was so weak that I had to stop and rest at least three times!

It was then that I realized that if I had received the full units of chemotherapy that I had been recommended, my entire white blood cells would have been completely wiped out. Could you imagine?! If a small dose of chemotherapy, had lowered my white blood cells so drastically, what would have happened if I had taken a large dose? It could have been fatal for me.

I was only able to take four treatments of low dose chemotherapy during my ten-day stay, but I was given large doses of natural chemotherapy.

There was a special relationship developed between the nurses, the other cancer patients, their spouses and us. On several occasions, we all had prayer and devotion. We were all from different places in the U.S, such as Washington State, Texas, Connecticut, California, and, of course, New York. We were all there for the same reason, and that was to overcome cancer.

The nurses were caring, dedicated, and professional in their duties toward me. They did not make me feel like an outcast. I distinctly remember how friendly they were. Their mindset was all about keeping us positive and believing that we could beat cancer.

After my initial ten days, I returned to New York for one month, to give my body a chance to recuperate, before returning on my second trip for ten days of low dose radiation.

After chemotherapy and radiation, my largest tumor had shrunk to about a third of its original size. The smaller tumors could not be found at all! This was quite encouraging. I was eating better and feeling better. I was indeed optimistic because my next step was to return home to do the surgery to remove the remaining tumor. But, I encountered a problem.

It was necessary to find a surgeon who was willing to do my surgery. Unfortunately, after meeting with two doctors, they both turned me down. I was told that in the United States the procedure is to do surgery first, then followed by radiation treatments. Since I had already done radiation in Mexico, the doctors felt that I would bleed out during surgery. They did not want to take the risks.

So, I had no choice but to go back to Mexico. I made the decision, to leave the United States, where my health insurance was covered, to go to Mexico, which was not, necessarily the place I thought I would do surgery; and where my insurance was not accepted.

On my third trip to Mexico, I met the surgeon who would perform the subcutaneous double mastectomy, to remove the remaining tumor as well as the breast tissue and lymph nodes that were affected. Being hospitalized in Mexico was itself an adventure.

Adventures with Lenny: Cancelling Cancer

There was an episode in the hospital, which I will never forget. The doctor sent a car to pick us up from the hotel. We then journeyed for about an hour through many unfamiliar parts of the city until we came upon a small building. This was the hospital where my surgery would take place.

As we entered the hospital, I saw them place big silver chains on the inside doors. My husband and I looked at each other. Although this act was odd, we reasoned that this area of Mexico seemed to require high security. They wanted to ensure that no uninvited persons could get in, but neither could we get out!

Lenny and I scrutinized the inside of the hospital, as we were escorted to a waiting room that was brightly lit with a sunroof, and decorated with many green, leafy plants.

After a short wait, I was escorted to my room where I stayed until the surgery. There were two beds in my room, so my husband was right across from me.

Have you ever been in a hospital where you were the only patient? Well, this was my experience for a while. This was weird, but I was okay with it because, the surgeon came highly recommended by my doctor who had already proven to be supportive, caring and reliable. And though it was strange being the only patient in that hospital for a while, I would not trade it for the world. Imagine I had 100% of the nurses and doctors' attention!

Emergency from the USA

I distinctly remember the day that they prepared me for the surgery. The plan was not to do a double mastectomy, as was prescribed in the United States. Instead, the plan was to do a double 'subcutaneous' mastectomy.

I was in the process of being prepared for my surgery when I was told that it would have to be postponed until the following day. There was someone, who had just been flown in, from the United States that was in a critical state, he needed immediate surgery. In fact, they asked me: "Would you please allow this man to take your place?" Of course, I agreed!

I later learned that he had colon cancer, it was said that his American doctors had given up on him, and his wife brought him to Mexico, as a last resort.

Finally, my time came again, and I was wheeled into the operating room, to endure a five-hour surgery. When I regained consciousness, I saw my husband, sitting across from me. Lenny was quite relieved to see me awake. He told me that my body was freezing cold when I was brought back to the room. Lenny also said to me that after I was in surgery for about four hours, he became concerned, so he went to check.

Lenny recounted how he just looked through a glass window in the door, while they operated. He was so scared for me, and it seemed like an eternity. Lenny said that he was in deep prayer because he was handicapped by anxiety when he realized that he couldn't physically help me.

The doctors and nurses came by, to see me after my surgery. They made sure that my recovery was going as expected. They monitored me for any swelling, bleeding or blood clots. I had some slight discomfort, and my arm was numb for a while, but overall, I had no significant pain or bleeding.

I was hospitalized for six days. I did not have to worry about food, most of the time. I was hooked to an intravenous bag. But, Lenny, my husband went six days with very little to eat, there was no way for him to leave the hospital. Lenny had a bag of mixed nuts, a loaf of bread, an 8-ounce piece of cheese, and a gallon bottle of water. This is what he rationed for the six days while we were there.

Soon, it was time to return to the United States. My doctor was concerned, he said: "You've got to go back to the U.S and hope to find an oncologist who will work with you and who will continue your treatment."

I was told to continue with my low-dose chemotherapy as well as the natural remedies. My tumors were gone, but my margins were not cleared. So, just in case there were any lingering cancer cells, I needed to continue treatment for six months for total recovery.

As I conclude this chapter, I must tell you that Mexico holds a lot of treasured moments for me. It was such a pleasant experience, from the time I spoke to Dr. S.V., to meeting him and finally, being treated by him!

The most important thing, I want to say about this doctor, is that his low dose chemotherapy and low dose radiation treatments, along with natural chemotherapy worked for me. Somehow, this method helped maintain my body's immune system, while it destroyed the cancer cells. It is my greatest hope that one day, low dose treatments, will be an option in the United States.

After arriving back home, I was blessed when my Gynecologist recommended an oncologist who agreed to continue my treatments. She reviewed my medical records from Mexico and worked with me during my six months of precautionary maintenance.

While doing this, I continued with natural remedies, many of which I will share later. This plan destroyed the possibility of any lingering cancer cells. The process for me was complete.

Chapter 9

Dare to Prove God

"Every evening I turn my worries over to God.
He's going to be up all night anyway."

-*Mary C. Crowley*-

Misconceptions about Cancer

Several people at different times asked me:
"Why did cancer happen to you when you were the one who practiced a vegetarian lifestyle?"

Such questions made me feel bad. I didn't know what precisely caused my situation, but their questions gave me an opportunity to answer. I tried to help them understand that being healthy is much more than being a vegetarian or having proper nutrition. There is so much more to a healthy lifestyle. So even though I might have been a vegetarian, there were other healthy principles I needed to practice. Furthermore, no one, not even medical doctors know all the contributing factors that may lead to cancer.

It could be hereditary, injury, environmental, dietary, or many other contributing factors.

Staying healthy also entails getting adequate rest. I admit, I was not getting enough sleep, I was staying up late at nights taking care of my clients' needs, while I held a fulltime job during the day. It took a lot out of me. Now, as I look back, I was not doing myself any favors by neglecting my sleep. I implore you, dear reader, to get proper rest and take care of yourself.

Possible Contributing Factors to my Breast Cancer

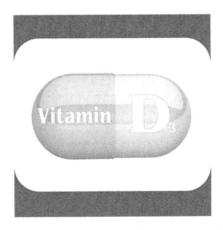

In addition to the contributing factors mentioned in the previous section, I want to mention that it is essential to get enough sunshine. That's why I want to talk about vitamin D3. I heard a doctor say that a lack of vitamin

D3 may cause different types of cancers, including breast cancer. I had never checked my vitamin D3 before this and was not aware that my D3 levels were precariously low.

Accountants and other office workers face this disadvantage. Many of us work in offices sealed off from sunlight. In my case, I spend approximately ten hours, each day working in an air-conditioned room with absolutely no sunlight.

Bear in mind, that our bodies particularly our skin, need to be exposed to the sunlight to make vitamin D3. There are so many cold months and days that we tend not to make enough vitamin D3. This is all the more reason why supplementation may be necessary.

A simple blood test can check your vitamin D3 levels. The normal range should be, between 20 to 50 ng/ml, and my result was 8! Once I discovered how low my vitamin D3 levels were, my doctor immediately had me take 5000 IUs per day until I got my levels up. It makes common-sense to have your doctor check your vitamin D3 levels.

To God be the Glory

God does not heal us from our sins and sickness, just to keep us alive or because we are better than somebody else. God will heal us to bring honor and glory to Him and to help somebody to increase their faith in Him. Do you agree?

And even if you don't survive your crucible in the physical, if you have the spiritual healing, eternal life is promised to you.

The Little, Sweet Things

It's not out of the ordinary to feel as if you've lost control because of a diagnosis. You may not be able to control the situation, but you can control yourself. I tried my best to keep my mind positive and active. I kept on humming songs and repeating psalms to myself all throughout the day. When I took my shower, I was thanking God for every organ in my body. I always found things for which I was thankful. When someone asked me how I was doing, I kept my smile and always answered. "Great!"

I believe that it is the simple things that we should be most grateful. They are the minutiae that hold the larger affairs of life together. Think about the ability to breathe involuntarily while asleep. How about the ability to chew your food, and all other unmentioned mercies of our Creator?

Life Lessons learned during Cancer

Not only are the privileges of life significantly necessary, whether they are simple or not, but everything in your experiences is meant to teach lessons, to help you win your battles. One lesson I learned during my struggle is, to always remain positive. I would visualize myself being healthy and free to talk about it. I strived to reflect health and happiness.

You are a unique creation and were made to be healthy, wealthy and secure. Additionally, the Bible says that you are "fearfully and wonderfully made." If you want your health to improve, do something; explore all your options; dare to prove God by taking action; The power to choose is a gift that the creator has made available to all.

Good health is a testimony to the goodness of God. It is to everyone's benefit to strive for good health. When we are not experiencing good health, it is imperative to work in harmony with God's plan. After all, God created us, and He is more than capable of restoring our body, mind, and spirit.

PART 3

APPRECIATE THE LOVE

AND SUPPORT

Chapter 10

A Lesson in Courage

"I learned that courage was not the absence of fear, but the triumph over it. The brave man is not he who does not feel afraid, but he who conquers that fear." - Nelson Mandela

Do not Give Up on Victory

As long as you have life, never give up on yourself. Your story may be so inspiring and compelling that it may transform someone else life!

Fear and doubt will sometimes cause a person to lose out on the benefits of faith. The moment you allow doubt to enter your belief system, you are entertaining defeat and giving up on your victory. For me, it took this devastating experience with cancer to make me dig deep within myself and lean on my belief. My faith and strength helped carry me through this challenge.

Family and Friends

Sickness can be a lonely venture. It's a time of uncertainty, and doctors cannot be definitive about a cure. The need for support from family, friends and the community, cannot be over-emphasized.

My family and friends were emotionally available for me. Knowing that many of them were there emotionally was also as important as them being there physically. I don't know what I would have done without them. I had so many telephone calls and well-wishers that I could not record them all. Just knowing that people were thinking about me, helped me stayed focused on my fight. Some of my clients kept telling me: "We need you to be around for a long time."

The words I wanted to hear most from my family and friends was that everything would be okay, that I had a good chance of surviving cancer. In retrospect, I recognize that inspiring words and positive affirmations made me feel empowered and courageous, like a winner!

Cancer can happen to anybody. It doesn't care who you are, where you are from, your profession, societal status, your religion or spirituality, it does not matter.

"Breast cancer alone kills some 458,000 people each year, according to the World Health Organization, mainly in low- and middle-income countries. It has got to be a priority to ensure that more women can access gene testing and lifesaving preventive treatment, whatever their means and background, wherever they live."[13]
-Angelina Jolie-

The Courage to Kill Cancer

You can be strong and courageous as you successfully fight any cancer. I am living proof. If you are a cancer patient, you must seek ways to combat. If you are not diagnosed, you must live healthily and stay that way.

My grandmother had stomach cancer. She always called it the 'Big C.' Fear causes people not to want to mention its name. There is a story in the Bible about one fearful servant that depicts how fear can hinder progress.

The master in this parable gave talents to three of his servants. They were to invest while he was away. One servant got five talents, the second two, and the third got one talent. Upon the master's return, the

---

[13]Jolie. A. My Medical Choice, by Staff Reporter. (2013, May 14), paragraph 16. Retrieved from http://www.destinyconnect.com/2013/05/14/my-medical-choice-angelina-jolie-2013-05-14/

servants with five and two talents made a hundred percent profit by doubling their investment, but the servant with one talent had no increase and made excuses. He told his master that he was afraid and hid his investment in the earth. (Matthew 25:25 KJV).

While the first two servants received blessings and rewards, the last servant was pronounced wicked and lazy. His fear had him paralyzed. It caused him not even to try.

It takes courage to fight cancer. We must not allow fear to cause us to make excuses, stop trying, and give up. We must remember the promises of our master. Fear will cause us to forget that God has promised to help. We can only win when we release our fears, stay encouraged, and trust God to come through for us. I held on to these soothing words God's promise:

"Fear thou not; for I am with thee: be not dismayed; for I am thy God: I will strengthen thee; yea, I will help thee" (Isaiah 41:10 KJV)

The Courage Extended

When a person is sick, their family and friends are going through a tough time also. Remember that they still have daily responsibilities. They need encouragement as well. It was challenging at times, for them trying to help me meet my needs while attending to their own. I will always be humbled and grateful to my family and friends who have inspired me with the will to fight and the encouragement to win.

Chapter 11

Love is thicker than Blood

"Once someone said to me, 'I'll ride the waves with you till the storm calms,' and that meant a lot to me because I knew they would be with me no matter what."

- Arthur Unknown -

The Power of Love

Receiving unconditional love is like being handed a special gift during a serious illness. I was fortunate to experience the best care in the world from my husband, Lenny. He is my earthly hero. I don't know how he did all that he did, but he did everything.

Lenny was my prayer partner, my chauffeur, my nurse, my personal assistant, my administrative professional, my home attendant, my chef and my publicist!

He prayed with me, he drove me to the doctors, accompanied me to my appointments, he knew what information to record to report back to the doctor at my next appointment, he consoled our daughters, took care of our home, updated friends and family on my progress, he fed me, I was supported in every way.

Lenny exemplified the meaning of the wedding vow: "For better and for worse, in sickness and in health." He lived up to his promises, and this was instrumental in my turnaround. I'm blessed to be married to an extraordinary and supportive man. What if a person is not so blessed to have such a spouse? Then find a caretaker, a trusted friend, a significant person, because this is not only important, it is necessary.

You need someone who loves you to get through illness, not only for doctor appointments but the simple mundane things. Things like changing your clothes, preparing your prescribed meal plan, filling out health forms, asking the right questions on your behalf and connecting with healthcare practitioners.

You tend to get better treatment when the practitioners and doctors realize that you are not alone. Someone who has your best interest at heart has your back and is willing to get involved with your care. You need someone to keep your mind on the real possibility that you may be around for a long time when others think you may not.

Love and Support

Scars from cancer can make you look ugly and feel the worse you have ever felt, but the support from your loved ones makes you realize that there is no shame, you will never have to fight alone, powerful prayers are going up on your behalf, and life is worth fighting for.

Support from loved ones keeps your 'mojo' and joie de vivre intact! Having a positive attitude is exactly what you will need to speed your recovery as you battle your cancer demon.

Show Gratitude

What is there to be grateful for, during cancer, you might ask? There are many things to be thankful for at all times. In our pursuit of the 'American dream,' it is very easy to overlook the important people and processes that impact our lives.

For example, I had long needed to find someone to help me organize my business, and once I began to pray about it, God sent me Yzamar Bravo. Yzamar is one of the most competent professionals I have ever worked with. She does a fantastic job of keeping me organized and helps me follow up with my clients. Yes! Yzamar has been a dream come true, in my life. When you sincerely pray for things, keep your thoughts positive, and show gratitude, then the Lord will answer.

Life is like climbing a mountain; you ascend to different levels, one after another until you reach the summit. After you accomplish one dream, you then move on to another. When we achieve our goals, it's great to show gratitude by serving and helping others.

Love Is Not Selfish

It is said that:

"God is love." (1 John 4:8 KJV).

Jesus Christ manifested His love for humanity, by dying on a cross for us. The thickest blood of all was shed in that selfless act of love. His love is perfect, and unconditional. Although I know that I must show gratitude and appreciation for the personal sacrifices that many have made for me during my illness, knowing that Jesus laid down His life makes me more thankful than ever.

Cancer can make a person feel depressed and secretive about their illness. But when people treat you nicely, they light up when they see you, and you sense acceptance in their eyes, they care about your well-being, something happens deep within your spirit that gives you the will to go forward. It's a feeling that is hard to express, but it happened to me.

I did not have to hide. My hairdresser, Mumbie

Jack-Mcrae and I went out and bought a wig in anticipation of me losing all my hair from the chemotherapy, but I did not need it. My hair did not fall out because of the low dose chemotherapy that I used. Regardless of my situation, even if my hair did fall out, or when I was virtually skin and bone, my veins had turned dark, I felt weak, my body had looked old and haggard from sickness, I did not have to hide. This was Ann Marie, warts and all!

I was not nervous about sharing my illness. I laid down at night believing that this was a temporary situation that will end well.

My support system was my husband Lenny, my daughters, Nyala and Aletea, my Mom and siblings, my in-laws, my great friends, Marlene Robinson, Judy Brown, Eslyn Phillip-Carter, and Cheryl Ann Jordan. My caretakers Janet Holmes and Gwen Shorter, my doctors, and many pastors and church family. What an amazing network! I owe thanks and gratitude to them all.

Chapter 12

Letting Go to Let God

"Now therefore stand and see this great thing,
which the LORD will do before your eyes."
-1 Samuel 12:16 (King James Version)

Reasons to Let Go During Cancer

During these crucial times you may have to let go, but letting go is never an option unless the one you are yielding to, can do a better job than you.

This battle with cancer demanded my all. I tried every regimen that I learned: ionized alkaline water, the barley grass green juices, walking, exercising and so much more. Cancer demanded the best of me and, yet I knew it would take more than what I had to give, to assure victory. So, I reached out, and I reached up. I reached out to those around me, like my doctors and lifestyle educators. And I reached up to the Creator:

"I will lift up mine eyes unto the hills, from whence cometh my help. My help cometh from the LORD..." – Psalms 121:1-2 KJV

Man alone is not enough but God alone is always sufficient. Divine intervention is real, and I had to let go to let God work on my behalf.

I want to motivate people diagnosed with cancer, to trust God to keep His promises. An important aspect of my experience was my strong faith and belief in the promises of God. I recall a pastor reassuring me that it was entirely okay to wonder why this had happened to me, to ask God why this would happen to someone who ate well. However, he said: "Don't get stuck asking, Why me?" Instead, ask: "What lesson are you trying to show me, Lord?" I would often ask myself: *What's my silver lining in this experience?* These questions allowed me to let go of the worrying, give thanks to God, and keep going on with my day.

Dear reader, may this book encourage you to have that trust and faith in God because He can hear you and you must first believe. Remember the biblical story about the woman with the issue of blood? For twelve long years, she suffered from chronic bleeding, she spent all her money on the physicians of the day, but she only grew worse. One day, she heard that Jesus, the miracle worker, was coming to town. So, she decided to risk it all; she made her way through the madding crowd, the pulling and pushing must have been overwhelming. But the faithful woman kept her eyes on the prize, Jesus! As she approached him, she fell to her knees and grabbed for the hem of his garment. Miraculously, she recovered. Jesus felt her little, special touch and said to her that by faith she had been healed. I cannot over-emphasize the virtues of faith.

Work with Your Doctor

Let me express how crucial it is to understand that it is okay to work along with your doctor and with their consent using a natural plan as well. This may seem obvious, but it is not always so.

I was working along with lifestyle educators, and they had cautioned me about chemotherapy and radiation because of the known side effects of those treatments on the body. Medical doctors rely on the standard medical protocols of the day, they are scientific, and some may not accept the idea of herbal or natural protocols. They may also be skeptical about the role of faith in a person's healing since it is an intangible that cannot be seen or tested. However, they are aware that a positive frame of mind works wonders on the body. An old Trinidadian proverb says, "common-sense before book sense," I felt inspired to take the best that both worlds had to offer:

chemotherapy and radiation in low dose amount along with natural protocols. If you meet with resistance from your doctors about your decision, find a way to work with them. You cannot do this without them.

Keep in mind that although I used low dose chemotherapy and radiation, it did not guarantee my survival. I also used many natural remedies and protocols. So, remember that God has given wisdom to doctors to implement healing on their patients, but He has also given us powers to execute His plan in our lives.

I do believe that natural remedies played a massive part in my recovery, I also think that we cannot do without our medical doctors. Were it not for the fact that I had my body scanned; I would not have known just how fast the cancer was growing. Medicine does not mean we should rule out natural. The two are not mutually exclusive.

Let me share this story:

I had a friend who was also diagnosed with breast cancer. To my knowledge, she chose not to take any chemotherapy or radiation. She decided only to use natural remedies.

I shared with her how God led me through my crucible and how I prevailed, using low dose chemotherapy and radiation, and high amounts of natural remedies. I had hoped she would try it. However, she did not.

One day she called me and shared that she was walking a mile every day. She said that she was also very optimistic. She believed that she was cured. She even sounded like it that day.

She asked me if I knew a place where she could go to do more cleansing and rebuilding of her body. Eventually, she found a place that she liked, but when she got there, it didn't take long for her caretaker to recognize that something was very wrong and ordered her to go to the doctor immediately.

She was taken straight to the hospital. Her cancer was so critical and widespread, and there was nothing the hospital could do. What a shock! About a week later, she succumbed to the disease. This news was tough and sad for her family, friends and me.

From Hopelessness to Healing

Desperate times call for courage and stamina. You can be mentally and spiritually strong even in the face of ill health.

The Bible speaks of a man who was lying at the side of a pool for thirty-eight years (John 5:5-15). He was lame, homeless and hopeless. Every year he waited for the moving of the water by some miraculous agent. But, he could never get someone to help him into the water, everyone who could move was always ahead of him. Then, at this man's highest point of hopelessness, the Savior came by.

The first question Jesus asked this man was, "would you like to be made whole?' The lame man immediately began to utter excuses that he has no one to help him get into the water. Jesus wanted him to readjust his attitude and shift his focus from what he could not do on his own, to what he could do through Christ Jesus.

Sometimes in life people may trample you, they may run ahead of you because they can move faster than you, they may ignore you, they may treat you wrong, and it hurts, I know. But, take courage. Think of that pool as your freedom, let go of the hopelessness and let the Savior give you that healing.

"Arise!" Jesus said to the surprised, confused man. Take up your bed and walk." The Bible said, immediately the man "took up his bed and began to walk." How was that possible? First, he was lame, and could not move for thirty-eight years, then in a split second, he was walking with his bed, probably on his head! How awesome it is to know that "all things are possible through Christ Jesus!"

Maybe just as awesome as the way I felt when I found out my cancer was gone. I wanted to leap from the floor into the air! Freedom from cancer means, being free to accomplish more goals and to get more awareness out. Like choosing to write this book, because God has given me the freedom to do it.

We all can choose to allow our freedoms in life to motivate us. If you have the privilege of good health currently, make the right decisions and be motivated to remain that way. In my opinion, health is our only real wealth!

Chemotherapy: The Gift and the Curse

The experience of chemotherapy is unique, and it is a classic case of being between a rock and a hard place. It is an experience that many never live through, but those who do will always remember. As the chemotherapy snakes through your veins, you pray that it will destroy those horrible cancer cells, but you are very concerned about the poisonous effects on your good cells.

Before you can count from one to one hundred, drowsiness steps in and many times you doze off. Then it's done, as you get up and walk you sometimes feel exhausted and nauseous. It is something you did not want to take, but you did anyway.

The common-sense part of this experience is to remember to do the necessary things to rebuild those good cells and your immune system before and after chemotherapy.

Hope conquers the Effects of Cancer

Weak health requires strong hope. One way I fought to combat cancer's ugliness was to overpower it with the beauty of hope.

This hope meant maintaining a winning attitude no matter what. Winning against cancer was also about being observant. I took note of the reactions of other patients. Some people chose not to talk or share their feelings, and I distinctly remember one patient who received chemotherapy in the same room with me, she did not want to hear about or see her blood reports. Her husband spoke with her doctor, but she did not want to know the results. I observed the sadness on her face and was determined to be the opposite.

I wanted to hear what my doctors had to say, I wanted others to pray daily for me, I wanted to end up on the winning side of cancer, so I shared my sickness and remained hopeful.

While some view cancer as an unpardonable death sentence, I needed to begin thinking of it as, a lousy sickness from which I could get a stay of execution. Then, use my time after the disease to live a great life of thanksgiving, bringing awareness, motivating and inspiring others. Yes, cancer is worth conquering!

I will Survive Breast Cancer!

"You think I'd crumble? You think I'd lay down and die? Oh no, not I, I will survive. Oh as long as I know how to love, I know I'm still alive. I've got my life to live, and I've got all my love to give. And I'll survive, I will survive"[14]

If you are currently a cancer patient, know that with much optimism and decisive actions, you stand a better chance of survival. Rearrange only one word. Instead of thinking: *will I survive?* You must say it like a champion: I WILL SURVIVE! Even though, Gloria Gaynor, the celebrated American disco singer was singing about a man in her famous international 1978 hit song: 'I Will Survive.' her lyrics are an equal rebuke to cancer.

View obstacles in life as bumps in the road, as challenges to be faced. Each obstacle solved, helps to strengthen and better prepare you to meet another, while leading you closer to achieving your goals.

Use your own God-given common-sense before making every decision. Accept your situation in life and begin to fight to change it.

---

[14] Gaynor, Gloria. Lyrics. I Will Survive

Healing Begins in the Mind

It has been said that healing begins in the mind. I asked. I believed. I received. Thank God!

I knew in my mind that I was not ready to die. I had so much I still wanted to accomplish. I wanted to see my girls finish college and get married, spend more time with my grandchildren, buy my dream house. And oh, I wanted to build my business and earn my first one million dollars in my lifetime. So, you see, dying was nowhere on my to-do list!

In the next few chapters, I am going to tell you what it means to maintain purpose for your life.

Part 4

MAINTAIN THE

PURPOSE FOR YOUR

LIFE

Chapter 13

Using Common Sense

"Knowledge is a powerful tool, but what is knowledge if not implemented? I am so thankful for the knowledge of the medical and natural doctors that worked with me. It was the combination and implementation that helped me survive." -Ann Marie Fraser-

Strike Back Against Cancer!

One doctor I met in Mexico told me: "Some people can handle the effects of the treatment better than others. You don't seem to be one of them, so remember to keep your white blood cells up".

I made a strike against cancer. My goal was to keep my white blood cells as high as possible so that they could fight the disease for me. I always asked for a copy of my blood results before every treatment. Then, I took steps to build up my immune system on a daily basis, using natural protocols in between treatments. This made so much common-sense to me.

Employ Better Lifestyle Habits

Another strike against cancer was implementing better lifestyle habits. Cancer is an enemy, and therefore you should combat that enemy from the moment you become aware of it.

Having cancer made me more keenly aware of what should go into my body and also what should be discarded. Things to be eliminated are alcohol, smoking, meats, greasy foods, sugars, acidic forming foods like white flour, white macaroni, white bread, and beverages like soda.

What I always heard was that cancer thrives in an acidic environment. Conversely, cancer cells are starved in an alkaline environment. Dr. Otto H. Warburg was awarded the Nobel Prize in medicine in 1931, and

"Dr. Warburg has made it clear that the root cause of cancer is oxygen deficiency, which creates an acidic state in the human body. Dr. Warburg also discovered that cancer cells are anaerobic (do not breathe oxygen) and cannot survive in the presence of high levels of oxygen, as found in an alkaline state."[15]

It's about common-sense education. Being responsible for our health involves making lifestyle changes, doing what's best for our bodies and doing it consistently.

A Common-Sense Synergy

Again, I want to be clear that, I did not rule out medicine. I used what I call, a common-sense synergy, to help me fight against cancer. For emphasis, its definition is worth restating. It can also be described as a combination of different things. According to Business Dictionary Synergy is defined as:
"A state in which two or more things work together in a particularly fruitful way that produces an effect greater than the sum of their individual effects."[16]

---

[15]Warburg, O.H. The Root Cause of Cancer, Ganodermareview, Nobel Prize Winner. Retrieved from
https://sites.google.com/site/ganodermareview/the-root-cause-of-cancer

[16] Synergy Definition, *Business Dictionary.com*

In the same way, I used a combination of four things to help me fight cancer with my faith in God leading and guiding over all four:

1. Medicine
2. Natural Protocols
3. Support from Family & Friends
4. Positive Attitude

The first thing I did was pray to God because I believe in prayer. Prayer opens the floodgates of heaven. I want to motivate that person who might one day be diagnosed with cancer, to trust in God to keep His promises. To know that trust and faith in God, as small as a mustard seed, can move mountains.

"If ye hath faith as a grain of mustard seed, ye shall say unto this mountain, remove hence to yonder place, and it shall remove; and nothing shall be impossible unto you." Matthew 17:20.

He says that he can heal you and you must first believe that He can.

Do not rule out medicine. I used chemotherapy and radiation in low doses. Work with your doctors. As you are working under your doctor's care, you need to know that you are also working under God's care, for He, has given wisdom and knowledge to the doctors.

I also used natural protocols, which will be

shared later in this book. I employed several common-sense protocols that I learned from lifestyle educators who, in my opinion, truly understand the effects of natural health principles on the body.

It is also important to recognize the role of supportive family and friends, as well as the benefits of a positive attitude, which I aimed to keep all the way through. I sincerely believe that I am alive today because of my common-sense synergy!

Each part of the synergy plays a unique role in affecting the outcome. One cannot be substituted for the other. For example, you cannot double up on medicine and think that it will substitute for the support of family and friends. All the elements are necessary to help you be better prepared to fight cancer.

When you have good doctors, it helps build your confidence against cancer. When you have positive encouragement and support, it makes you more self-assured. When you employ natural health principles and positivity, it aids in your recovery and strengthens your resolve. When God gives you blessings, and you see progress, it lifts your spirit. Remember, fighting cancer is like being in a battle; you are undertaking a battle for your life, you need to have the confidence of David against Goliath!

My Temple is not made for Cancer

God recognizes our bodies as sacred, in fact, like a temple. He sees us as His most beautiful creation, and He values us dearly. It is difficult to see ourselves as sacred when cancer is present, and our body is fighting against itself. Yet God wants us to be made whole:

"Know ye not that your body is the temple of the Holy Ghost which is in you, which ye have of God, and ye are not your own?... Therefore, glorify God in your body, and in your spirit, which are God's." 1 Corinthians 6:19 KJV)

He places a responsibility on us to preserve our bodies in the best condition possible, then share that knowledge with others.

Cancer Therapy

Helping others was a form of therapy for me. I began to feel better about myself when I realized that I could bring tremendous inspiration and hope to those coping with cancer. Strangely I am thankful for my survival experience. It has made me stronger and wiser and has filled me with a sense of peace. I guess that is what the scriptures meant when it said:

"And the peace of God, which surpasseth all understanding, shall keep your hearts and minds..." Philippians 4:7 (KJV)

And now it brings me great joy as my greatest desire is to help and encourage others to overcome and live healthier lives.

Chapter 14

The Fight Continued

"It's about focusing on the fight and not the fright."

-Robin Roberts

Cancer is real! My God is real!

Dealing with breast cancer and its accompanying stress is hard. Ironically, stress itself, increases the risk of cancer. Throughout my struggles, I kept reminding myself: Why should I be afraid when I know my God is real!

Cancer is a physical and spiritual struggle. It tested my faith and challenged my patience. By acknowledging that God is all-powerful, I was willing to search for deeper meanings, while applying His principles to my situation.

We can all take comfort from the conviction of

the Apostle Paul who said that he could do all things through Christ. God can perform a miracle in your future, so don't be afraid or hesitant to continue the fight, no matter how bad it gets. There is no mountain He cannot climb, no boundaries He cannot cross, His solution is infinite and is far reaching beyond human intellect. So, decide right now in your mind to live your life to the fullest, regardless of how severe life gets, even if it is cancer.

Sacrifice for Survival

Another fundamental attitude to develop during the fight is the will to make consistent sacrifices for survival. My objective was to be around long after my cancer was gone. This required my 24/7 vigilance. It meant doing everything I could and accepting everything that others could do for me.

Lift Your Thoughts Higher

We can achieve anything, as long as our goals are in harmony with the will of God. We must lift our thoughts higher. Think positive and control negative thoughts.

You have to:

"Feed your faith and starve your doubts to death."[17] – Debbie Macomber

There can be no progress without personal sacrifice. The question is, what are you willing to give up to accomplish your goals? What new habits are you willing to adopt?

God doesn't stop halfway. There is no quitting with Him. He does not leave a task undone. Cancer is the most significant fight of your life, do not be afraid to fight for your life. The battle will continue but while it does maintain vital interactions.

---

[17]Macomber, Debbie - Quote

Chapter 15

Vital Interactions And Maintaining Intentions

"The first half of life is spent mainly in finding out who we are through seeing ourselves in our interaction with others."

- Dr. June Singer

Victory is in Your Path

Many times, there will be people in your life who will wish to see you fail, but there will always be people who want to uplift you. These are the people with whom you want to stay in close contact. You will also meet new people on your journey, who will point you in the right direction. I have come across individuals who I know without a doubt God has placed in my life for essential interactions.

Take a moment and recall the people who have had the most significant impact on your life. Maybe it's a great teacher who helped you realize you could achieve, perhaps a parent who unconditionally loved you, maybe a mentor who encouraged your dreams and aspirations. Who are those people that have inspired greatness in you? Those connections are vital to your success.

It's a basic human instinct for us to want to be successful at something. Whatever it is, you should work hard at achieving your goals every day. But you should include yet another goal: to be generous with your love and with your time. When you share those gifts, you're strengthening vital relationships and forming new friendships.

Very often, friendships are developed through adversity. I formed many new friendships because of my sickness, and I cherish them. Some of my new friends are cancer survivors with whom I felt an automatic connection because they knew what I have been through.

You may also find that family members, friends, coworkers, or business associates, sometimes, react to you differently after a cancer diagnosis. There may be a level of awkwardness, moments of uncomfortable silence or heavy pauses. Remember your loved ones are also going through shock, disbelief, and confusion, having to adjust to your illness. It may be that they have never had to deal with the real possibility that their loved one could die or it may create some uneasiness for them when faced with a reflection of their mortality.

Communication is Vital

Sometimes, what you think is just a time-consuming conversation can save somebody's life. Communication is important, and connections are invaluable, there is a difference between the two. Communication is an exchange of information, via a conversation, technology, or literature. A connection is about reaching someone on a visceral level, and it is a deep interaction of feelings, an exchange of emotion.

Communication is a relatively continuous process, whether you know it or not you are doing it even now with this information, either passively or actively. Real connections are rare, like finding your soul-mate!

I implore you that if you are ever diagnosed with any form of cancer, do not keep it a secret and try to go through it alone. Connect with people as much as you can to help you fight cancer. If you are blessed to have and find vital connections, cherish them even after you survive.

Maintaining Intention

"If God can cause the blind man to see, if He can cause the lame man to walk, if He can raise Lazarus from the dead; then certainly, He can rid a body of cancer cells. And with that second chance, let the intentions be to keep on encouraging as many people as possible."

-Ann Marie Fraser, cancer survivor.

The Power of Your Intentions

In my estimation, no other disease that plagues the human body has more fear and suffering attached to it than cancer. Not only does it drain your finances, but it can also sap the energy of the patient and their family. The intention is to survive and live to encourage others, but often the mind of the patient gets fixated on the problem rather than on a solution.

Wishful thinking alone will not work nor make healing a reality. Keeping your fingers crossed hoping for luck will not make sickness go away. It takes hard work, and you can do it. My grandmother, Annie Kinsale, always said to me "There is no such thing, as something for nothing." You will have to give up some things to attain your desires and good health.

The mind is the most powerful weapon we have. You would be surprised to know that healing begins in the mind. It must be kept clear of worry and stress. Maintain your intention to live by taking affirmative action and giving praises to God.

Learn how to straighten your question mark into an exclamation mark, 'As a man thinks so is he!' So, maintain positive intentions. Know that each time you fret and worry, cancer spreads more and more. Shut the door on pessimism and open the door to optimism. Here's how you turn a question mark into an exclamation mark:

Instead of asking: Why am I going through this? Say: Why not me!

Instead of asking: How am I going to deal with this? Say: I am not alone!

Instead of asking: Where am I going to find the money? Say: God will supply all my needs!

Instead of asking: Am I putting my family through stress? Say: This too shall pass!

Instead of asking: Will I remain attractive to anyone? Say: I will be unique to that someone!

Instead of asking: Am I going to die? Say: I am healed! Finally, say, thank you, Jesus!

Chapter 16

Strange Goodbyes

"Cancer may have started the fight, but I will finish it."-gotcancer. org.

"Time is shortening. But every day that I challenge this cancer is a victory for me...

~ Ingrid Bergman

Big Smiles and Goodbyes

Do you think it is easy to say goodbye to a part of oneself? It is a difficult thing. I was faced with saying goodbye, to both my breasts forever! My breasts were riddled with cancer cells, and a Double Mastectomy, was the medical recommendation. I was terrified, but after careful consideration, I decided to give a big smile and shout goodbye to those cancer cells in my breasts.

Overcoming a serious illness doesn't mean it's over. I know that may sound contradictory, but you're not out of the woods yet, you still have to do regular maintenance and keep on fighting. "The battle is not for the swift but for who can endure until the end."

I guess there is never a good time to have cancer. I remember when I discovered the tumor in my breast, my first thought was: "If it is cancer I will fight it!" Now that I have fought and beaten cancer, I don't consider myself a cancer survivor. I am a cancer survivor with a message.

One strong message is to learn everything you can about cancer receptors and preventing cancer from spreading. There are different breast cancer receptors: Tripple Negative, ER-Positive (estrogen hormone), PR-Positive (progesterone hormone), andHER2-positive. My doctor told me that my breast cancer receptor was the HER2-Positive.

"If your breast cancer is HER2-positive, it's more aggressive than other types of breast tumors... About one in every five breast cancers is HER2-positive. That means the cancer cells have more of a protein called HER2, human epidermal growth factor receptor 2. It causes these cells to grow and spread faster than the ones with normal levels of the protein..." [18]

---

[18] Blahd, W. Reviewed this article (2016, December 21). What Is HER2-Positive Breast Cancer? WebMD Medical Reference, Retrieved from

Many survivors worry that they have not said goodbye to cancer forever. They fear the possibility of a relapse. Anytime I feel pain; I wonder if my cancer is returning. It is not a great feeling, but doubt and anxiety will creep into your thoughts. Just smile, and shout goodbye to negativity! Pay particular attention to even the minutest changes in your body. You are the best person to know your own body, which can help you distinguish between normal physical changes and more serious symptoms. If you notice a sign report it to your doctor immediately.

The Remission Phase

Almost everybody gave me words of encouragement and quotes of inspiration. Many people shared herbal remedies with me, and others recommended that I visit natural lifestyle centers. But, the one thing that meant a lot was loved ones who prayed for me daily. I sincerely believe that man can appeal to God, by formal request, through prayer. In my case, God heard the petitions of their prayers and responded in my favor. He sent my cancer into remission!

In January 2009, my doctor told me that my cancer was in remission. Those words sounded like

https://www.webmd.com/breast-cancer/qa/what-is-her2positive-breast-cancer

music to my ear! I was so elated that I could not contain myself.

During the final six months of chemotherapy treatment, I would leave the doctor's office, wait for a bus, and often, I fell asleep on my way home. I felt drained from the side effects of the chemotherapy. But, this time was different. After hearing I was cancer-free, I left her office feeling a new burst of hope streaming through my veins. The creeping killer cancer could crawl no more.

There are two stages of remission.

"Partial remission means the cancer is still there, but your tumor has gotten smaller…, or in cancers like leukemia, you have less cancer throughout your body…, **Complete remission** means that tests, physical exams, and scans show that all signs of your cancer are gone. Some doctors also refer to complete remission as "no evidence of disease (NED)."[19]

Being in remission to me meant: No more chemotherapy, no more radiation, no more days in the hospital, no more pain. All signs of my cancer were gone, and there was no evidence of the disease! All I

---

[19] Ratini, M. Reviewed this article (2016, July 22). What Does Cancer Remission Really Mean? -WebMD, Retrieved from
https://www.webmd.com/cancer/remission-what-does-it-mean

was required to do was my annual Pet CT scan and a physical exam. I now have more time to accomplish goals and to help others.

Be Aware - Cancer Loves Complacency

Do not become complacent when in remission. Cancer loves to come back like a person who says with a vengeance "I'm back! And, there is no stopping me."

I have met people who were in remission for many years, yet this horrible disease came back and won. To enjoy good health after cancer, you must constrain thoughts of sickness and death. There is always a better way to think than continually believing that the end is around the corner. This does not mean that your mind won't ever stray on thoughts of death. However, think life without cancer.

What To Do While In Remission

1. Make a conscious effort to see that cancer does not return.
2. Focus on support and managing your newfound health and well-being.
3. Meet other cancer survivors, find out what they are doing and learn from them.
4. Do your regular annual checkup.
5. Do not stray from your healthy lifestyle. If you do,

return to healthy habits as quickly as possible.

6. Ask loved ones to hold you accountable for your actions.

7. Share your story and help inspire others.

Promote Health during Remission

One of my favorite authors wrote:

"Since *the mind and the spirit find expression through the body, both mental and spiritual vigor are in a great degree dependent upon physical strength and activity; whatever promotes physical health, promotes the development of a strong mind and a well-balanced character. Without health, no one can as distinctly understand or as completely fulfill his obligations to himself, to his fellow beings, or to his Creator. Therefore, the health should be as faithfully guarded as the character.*"[20]

---

[20] White, E.G. Education. Ch. 21. Study of Physiology, p. 195.1.

Part 5

YOU CAN DO ALL THINGS THROUGH CHRIST

Chapter 17

Your Health is Your Wealth

"Beloved, I wish above all things that thou mayest prosper and be in health, even as thy soul prospereth."
- 3 John 1:2 (King James Version)

Money can't buy Everything!

We all have hectic days, times when we are so busy, and there's not even time to eat! I have had many of those days, over an extended period. One day, a pastor friend said to me, "Ann Marie, if you love yourself you would stop doing that." Maintaining a healthy, balanced life is a challenge because we all get caught on the treadmill that is modern-day living, running to and fro with deadlines to meet or somewhere to be and things to do! But, I knew I had to stop working myself so hard and do better.

Money and financial security are essential to all of us, but let us not make the mistake of equating real success and happiness by merely having lots of money. Money may take care of our physical and social needs, but of what use would all that money be if, we didn't have good health along with it? It is my opinion that health is our true wealth!

I was doing so much that my life felt like a maze instead of being amazing. You know what they say about "all work and no play": it makes you very dull, indeed! Eventually, I sat down with my business coach to map out my priorities, to create some balance in my life.

Successful individuals are those with a well-rounded lifestyle. There must be synergy in the spiritual, physical and mental aspects of your life. These are your top priorities. If you desire real success and a long life with health and strength, then make it a priority to achieve a balance in your life. Maintain your equilibrium and strive to be temperate in all things.

The Race of Life: Be in It to Win It!

Pursuing spiritual growth will complement your material success. One Apostle said it this way:

'Know ye not that they which run in a race run all, but one receiveth the prize? So run, that ye may obtain.' (1 Corinthians 9:24 KJV).

Although many runners begin a race, only one receives the gold medal. You must run the race to win, and to win you must train, exercise, eat healthily, put in long hours, get adequate sleep and drink lots of good water. Winning the gold medal demands hard work, dedication, consistency, and discipline.

Prior to my diagnosis, I thought I was healthy because I was a vegetarian. Cancer made me come to realize that I needed to do more than eat right if I wanted the gold prize. I had to make a new beginning. Make a fresh start by taking better care of your body now. It's never too late to begin healthful living.

I adopted a healthier plan, and here are some things I determine to do daily to help me to win.

My Best Practices for Healthful Living

1. Trust in Divine power: Start the day with prayer. The Savior promised to heal and sustain me. I know without any doubt that it was the power of God that restored me from my disease. This recovery involved doctors, medicine, natural remedies, family, friends, caretakers, and much more. But, God has the last word. God's power is continually at work on man's behalf, and His power is open to you.

2. Practice deep breathing

I breathe in about 12 deep gulps of fresh air early every morning. I inhale through my nostrils, hold my breath for a second, and exhale through my mouth and sometimes nostrils. When I inhale, my stomach inflates. I try to take in as much air as possible. When I exhale, my stomach deflates.

Deep breathing helps to clear out the lungs, strengthen its capacity, and helps with respiratory problems. It supplies more oxygen which among many other things is needed to increase circulation of the blood while keeping the blood pure and moving. It is more beneficial to breathe open fresh air, rather than air from closed rooms. Fresh early morning air soothes the nerves and helps boost the immune system giving rise to stronger white blood cells. A healthier system is needed to destroy germs, bacteria, viruses, and fight cancer.

3. Drink lots of Ionized Alkaline Water.

I drink, daily, eight glasses of ionized, alkaline water, which I also use for cooking. Alkaline water has a higher pH level than regular drinking water. Because of this, it can neutralize acids in your body and has many other health benefits. Water rids the body of toxins, prevents dehydration, and is beneficial to the kidneys and urinary tract. Water helps facilitate proper digestion, helps strengthen the bowels, stomach, and liver.

Did you know that our brain is approximately 80% water, our bones are 22% water, and our body is 70% water?

Common-sense tells me that if I can get my water balance right, then it's a high possibility that I can get 80% of my brain right, 22% of my bones right, and 70% of my body right. Don't you agree? So, how do I drink eight glasses every day? I drink two glasses of ionized alkaline water in the morning, three glasses during the day, two glasses of water in the evening, and one before bed.

4. Physical Exercise.

In my younger days, I was a sports aficionado. Netball is a popular sport in my home country, Trinidad. However, I was horrified one day when I tried to bend down and realized I could not touch my toes. Now, I do stretch exercises in the morning, climb some short steps after lunch, and take brisk walks at least once per week. I also bounce 2-3 minutes on my rebounder daily. Exercise is essential for the body. Walking in the invigorating fresh air is helpful for the circulation of the blood. It has been said that "Perfect health demands perfect circulation." Physical exercise aids digestion and strengthens the heart.

5. Proper Sleep.

I get about six and a half hours of sleep every night, however, dear reader, if you can get more please do. Our busy, fast-paced society has made it increasingly difficult for us to get sufficient rest. The body regenerates new cells while we sleep, primarily between 10:00 pm and 2:00 am. We make ourselves sick by overworking, remember that proper rest is essential to the restoration of good health.

"Since the work of building up the body takes place during the hours of rest, it is essential, especially in youth, that sleep should be regular and abundant."[21]

---

[21] White, E.G. Education. Ch. 22. Temperance and Dietetics, p. 205.4

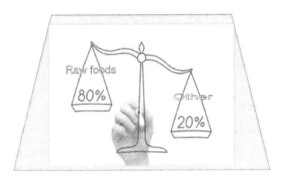

6. Eat Nutritious Meals

I eat as healthy as I can. It is important to choose organic foods whenever possible. Eat 80% raw foods and 20% cooked foods. Raw foods helped to starve my cancer cells. Eat more alkaline foods and less acid-forming foods. (See Additional notes on acid/alkaline forming foods)

The more I practiced a vegetarian lifestyle, the healthier I felt. Practice not to eat and drink at the same time. Drink your water or juice a half hour before meals or two hours after meals. Practice eating on time and avoid snacks between meals. As much as possible, I try to eat breakfast at 8:00 am, lunch at 1 pm, and my last meal at 6 pm. There's a funny saying: "Have breakfast like a King, lunch like a Prince and dinner like a Pauper!" It is better to indulge in your heaviest meal early and let your last meal be light.

Remove processed foods from your diet, like white flour, white rice, white macaroni, canned foods, etc. Eat more fruits and vegetables. Additionally, it is a good practice to fast. You may find by fasting for one or two meals, and by drinking only pure, alkaline water, it will reduce the burden on your digestive system. Despite the abundance of foods in our modern society, we should not eat and drink merely to satisfy unhealthy appetite cravings. Our bodies were designed to eat to live, not live to eat.

7. My Common Sense Education- 13 Protocols and Supplements

These are the 13 protocols I used:

See Additional notes for more information and details.

1) Ionized Alkaline Water

2) Ezzeac Tea

3) Cell Food Minerals

4) Barley Life Green Juice

5) Natural Chemotherapy

6) Anti-Oxidant Shots

7) Digestive Enzymes

8) Herbal Fiber Blend

9) Vitamin D3

10) IP 6 with Inositol

11) Colonics and Enemas

12) Hot and Cold Showers

13) Saunas

Chapter 18

You Can Do It Too

"No matter what you're going through, there's a light at the end of the tunnel and it may seem hard to get to it but you can do it and just keep working towards it and you'll find the positive side of things."

-Demi Lovato

Process without Cancer

You can overcome any obstacle in your way through God's power. But let's face it, to be successful in life you will need to go through a process. Success does not come overnight. A winner will tell you that the big difference between successful and unsuccessful individuals, is that one view failure as an opportunity to get it right next time, while the other views failure as FINAL. You can overcome your setbacks, and you can learn from other people's mistakes too.

I think of the people who have cancer, who may not get the opportunity to read this book, and who may die without getting a chance to apply my common-sense techniques to fighting and surviving cancer.

"My people are destroyed for lack of knowledge…" - -Hosea 4:6.

I think of the working mothers like myself, professional women, who work so hard daily taking care of their homes, husbands, children, bosses, pastors, and businesses, but somehow forget to take care of themselves.

I wish I could communicate to them the things they should be doing to avoid that horrible cancer diagnosis. I want to tell them to eat healthier and get annual checkups. I want to ask them to pay attention to their bodies. In the words of my Gynecologist:

"Any time you see anything strange or feel pain in your body, check it out." [22]

Dear readers, do not ignore the warning signs of pain, tenderness or even the slightest changes in your anatomy that are unfamiliar. I think of those who were diagnosed in the later stages of cancer and did not have enough time to fight back. I think of the younger generation who may not see a connection between what they put in their bodies and how it may affect their

---

[22] Comrie, Millicent - Center for Women's Health- Brooklyn, NY.

health in later years. I wish I could do more to bring awareness and to promote the message: "Prevention is better than Cure."

As a licensed Financial Professional, I conduct seminars on "how to manage your finances." My survival is a gift given to me by God, to share hope with those whose lives I might impact through my motivational speeches, my books or through my personal interaction. When it's all said and done, I believe that whatever state you find yourself you should never give up! As long as you can breathe, you must be hopeful.

Change your Mind and Change your Life!

While you are striving to succeed and to accomplish your goals, don't get so caught up in the desired outcome that you forget to enjoy the process. Remember, mistakes and missteps are for our personal development. How else would a baby learn to walk, if it did not fall a few times? Think about it, when a baby takes its first step, it is a step of faith. After a while, the baby knows, from experience that he or she will fall, but guess what, the baby steps out anyway! If a babe-in-arms can be fearless and have a winning attitude, what about you? If your habits are not helping you to win, let them go and pick up new ones.

Change your mind and change your life. Start today by letting go of who you think you are and see yourself as what you can be. Healthy, wealthy, and prosperous.

Pro-action vs. Reaction

Now that you are aware of the common-sense synergistic approach I used, and the other natural remedies I successfully used in my fight against breast cancer, you can decide for yourself if this is the approach you want to implement. The information I have shared about healthy living should be viewed as proactive, not reactive. According to the Malay proverb, *"Prepare your umbrella before it rains."* This fight against breast cancer, especially in women, takes knowledge and action. The choice is yours. Knowing your enemy will allow for a better defense against it.

30 Common-Sense Education Health Tips

1. Get to know all the facts about your cancer.
2. Learn about triggers and tumor markers.
3. Research the importance of a healthy white blood cell count.
4. Learn about the different stages of your cancer.
5. Research cancer survival rates.
6. Cleanse your body, then replenish it.
7. Consider using mineral flushes, coffee-enemas and colonics.
8. Take hot and cold showers
9. Enjoy nightly fiber intakes.
10. Consider liver, bladder and kidney flushes.
11. Use blood cleansers.
12. Eat healthy, whole or organic raw foods, as much as possible.
13. Implement an 80% raw and 20% cooked meals.
14. Drink and cook with ionized alkaline water.
15. Drink warm lemon water upon rising to help alkalize the body.
16. Use judiciously that which is healthful and nutritious.
17. Remove everything that is hurtful to your health.
18. No complicated recipes.
19. Give up junk foods.

20. Eat Simple, no more than 2 or 3 items at a time.
21. Have a green smoothie, a green salad or both daily.
22. Eat more alkaline food and less acid-forming foods.
23. Use vitamin and mineral supplements.
24. Reduce and/or eliminate your intake of sugars, flesh meats and processed foods.
25. Visit your healthcare practitioner regularly. Annual check-ups, may lead to early detection.
26. Cooperate with your doctors' requests, but don't be afraid to ask questions or make suggestions.
27. Seek information, always ask for a copy of your medical reports.
28. Inquire about low-dose chemotherapy and low-dose radiation. It may one day be an option.
29. Discuss using natural chemotherapy.
30. If things do not feel right, get a second opinion!

EPILOGUE

I defeated cancer by making common-sense decisions and using my Synergy plan of action. Ten years later, I remain free of the disease. My God deserves all the praise and glory!

I have accomplished a lot personally and professionally, and it feels great to be healthy. I challenge myself to live a healthier lifestyle in regards to diet, exercise, and nutritional supplementation. I've also changed a lot since that fateful Thanksgiving Thursday back in 2007 when my life was rudely interrupted by breast cancer. As a result, I do not doubt in my mind that my life has a Godly purpose.

I am blessed and highly favored. My experience with cancer and its treatment has taught me that this disease, is not necessarily a death sentence but it can become a life lesson! I've been burned by the fire, but I was not consumed.

My faith in an extraordinary God kept me steady. After dealing with cancer, you never know what the end of the road is going to be, and one thing I'm so thankful for is my wonderful husband, my daughters, my grandchildren, my relatives, and my friends.

My life has indeed changed. I have slowed down a bit, taking time to check on my family more often than before, and prioritizing as I work towards fulfilling my life's purpose. My mission through this book is to reach as many people as possible, with a positive message to trust in the healing power of Jesus Christ.

The prevailing notion is that cancer is a killer, especially in its later stages, but I decided that I did not want to live in fear of it. You can't fight any disease when you are afraid.

It is a known fact that when someone is faced with a schoolyard bully, they often become immobilized by irrational fear. It is when they talk themselves down from that high place of panic that they see clearly. Then, they realize that the bully breathes the same air they do and bleeds the same as they do. Facing your fears full-frontal is essential. I want to inspire others dealing with cancer to release their fear. It is better for courage and determination to take its place.

Whenever I see people striving for excellence in health, my heart skips a beat. Sincerely, I admire their tenacity and, the discipline it takes because I know that I am striving too. My sister-in-law Dorothy Richardson, whom I spent Thanksgiving with for many years, succumbed to cancer. Her death prompted me to work harder at finishing this book. It motivated a sense of greater urgency in me.

I know that God did not heal me so that I could relax and keep quiet. I learned so much from my time spent with Jan Holmes and Gwen Shorter; to my conversation with the late J.P, which led to my trips and adventures in Mexico with my husband Lenny; and to my successful recovery; I am determined to use my voice every opportunity I get.

Life has not been the same since my cancer diagnosis and treatment. I have become more focused. I now dedicate my life to spreading Common Sense Education about healthy lifestyle, financial health, and raising awareness about breast cancer among women in the United States, Canada, my birth country, Trinidad and Tobago, and the Caribbean in general. I believe that this book will reach far and wide around the world.

The most significant weapons in my arsenal against cancer were my faith in God, my God-given common-sense, dedicated medical and natural doctors, the love and support of my husband and family, and my synergy methodology. I am living proof of a miracle. I have received calls from numerous people over the past many years, and I am thankful that I have had the opportunity to give hope, faith, and comfort to them.

One doesn't win an Olympic gold medal after a few weeks of intensive training, most often it takes lifetime dedication and sacrifice. There is no bluffing one's way to success, and you must be willing to take the long, hard road. The Apostle Paul shared his formula for total success with Timothy:

'Meditate upon these things; give yourself wholly to them; that thy profiting may appear to all.'

(1 Timothy 4:15 NIV).

Final Words

In closing, I must say that the joy of living even if it's for one more day, outweighs my pain and suffering. Triumphing over my challenges makes life so much sweeter, so I think positive. I attribute my strength to prayer, faith, family, and seeking help with things that are beyond my expertise. Therefore, I do not worry about a relapse or death, that is God's decision, and I trust Him.

When I awake every morning, I give thanks and get out of bed with the intention to do the best that I can. I no longer run to and fro, like a headless chicken, in a frenzy, I pace myself, and I prioritize, I concentrate on living and earning so that I can be better prepared to help others financially. I might not have a million dollars yet, but either that million bucks is on its way, or I don't need it because I'm already successful beyond my wildest dreams. My health is my wealth.

"So many people spend their health gaining wealth. And then have to spend their wealth to regain their health." - AJ Reb Materi

Recovery does not happen overnight. It may take years of bad habits for the body to break down and it can take an even longer time for recovery. I implore you to pay attention to your body, follow the simple principles outlined in this book and put them into action. Do your part and allow God to do the rest. When something feels wrong, get tested immediately. Be determined to live healthier, and prevent or survive cancer, along with the other incredibly, brave human beings that have triumphed!

Additional Notes

Ionized Alkaline Water:

Cancer spreads in an acidic environment, so it's important to drink the right water which helps neutralize acid in the body.

This type of water can be made using an Ionizer machine. In my opinion, I use an ionizer that is far more effective than regular water filters. There is no substitute for the best when you desire good health, that is why I drink ionized, alkaline water as one of my secrets to maintaining good health. An ionizer machine can be hooked up to the kitchen sink and makes different types of water. I save money since I no longer need to buy bottled water for my home. The five types of water are strong acidic water, beauty water, clean water, three levels of alkaline drinking water, and strong alkaline water. You can obtain additional information about these types of water and their uses by sending an email to:

Info@annmariefraser.com
Or use referral ID# 1130267 when calling the manufacturer: 718-784-2199

www.useAlkalineWater.com

Ezzeac plus Cat's Claw Tea:

This tea is organic, natural, known as a blood purifier and the benefits of the herbs in the Ezzeac plus tea are numerous. I have been drinking it since 2008.

It contains six herbs which are:

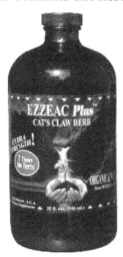

Burdock root-Burdock helps the body eliminate excess fluid assisting the kidney, liver, and overall digestive system. It is rich in the B and E vitamins also minerals which include potassium, phosphorus, iron, magnesium, zinc, silicon, cobalt, and chromium. Burdock Root is the main ingredient in the formula, and according to Dr. Bill Maclean, it is the most important.

The other five herbs in the tea are:
Sheep Sorrel Herb
Slippery Elm Bark
Turkish (Indian) Rhubarb Root
Watercress, and Cat's Claw Herb

For more information about the other five herbs contact: Company: Nature's Unique
Website: www.naturesunique.net

Email: Info@annmariefraser.com
ID#: ANNFRA, when contacting the manufacturer.

Cell Food Minerals:

"Cell food provides an incredible oxygen source and delivery system to the body at the cellular level…, in 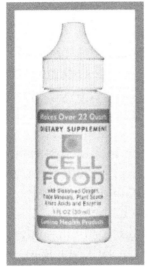 this formula are "Aerobic" proteins, 17 amino acids, 34 enzymes, 73 major and trace elements and deuterons, electrolytes and dissolved oxygen…,The inventor of cell food is Everett L. Storey, who was an author, physical chemist, microbiologist and humanitarian…, gives the following list of top seven cell food benefits:

Increased cellular respiration, metabolic efficiency catalyst, energy boosting properties, detoxifies the body deeply, balances the body metabolism, colloidal minerals, and special iconic form."[23]

Company: Nature's Unique
Website: www.naturesunique.net
Email: Info@annmariefraser.com
ID#: ANNFRA

---

[23] Cell food information adapted and Retrieved from
http://www.naturesunique.net/CELL_FOOD.HTM

The information referenced on this page is for informational purposes only. The opinions of the author(s) is/are not necessarily the opinions of The AIM Companies. Information provided should not be used for diagnosing or treating a health problem or a disease. Always consult a health practitioner prior to starting any health program.

Barley Life Powder:

"Barley grass juice — a wide spectrum of potent nutrients Research in the late 20th century revealed that young

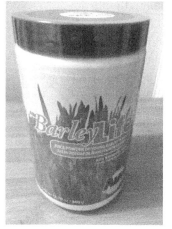

barley grass is the most nutritious of the green grasses. While barley has been used as a grain since ancient times, the value of barley as a grass was overlooked. Japanese researchers discovered that the young, green barley grass was an incredibly complete source of nutrition, containing a wide spectrum of vitamins, minerals, amino acids, proteins, enzymes, chlorophyll, and phytonutrients."

Fiber: In my opinion, the Aim herbal fiber blend is the best herbal cleanser on the market. It is a blend of many cleansing herbs including psyllium; provides both water soluble and insoluble fiber; helps maintain the digestive and eliminative tracks by removing toxins from the body with each bowel movement.

For More Information on the Barley Life Powder and
Herbal Fiber Blend contact:
The Aim Company at:
www.theaimcompanies.com
Referral ID#459855
1-800-456-2462

Examples of some Acid/Alkaline:

ACIDS	ALKALINE
Sugar	Lemmon
Stomach Juice	Saliva/Blood
Wheat	Dark Green Leaf's
Fowl	Vegetables
Egg	Millet
Meat	Quinoa
Cow Milk	Buckwheat
Corn Meal	Spelt
Wheat Bread	Amaranth
Canned Foods	Sea Water
Beer/Wine/Alcohol	Pancreatic Juice
Tobacco	Baking Soda
Other Grains	Soya Beans
Other Legumes	Lima Beans
Other Nuts	Almond
Grapes	Brazil/Chestnut
Grapefruit	Watermelon
Blueberries	Banana
Olives	Tofu
Pomegranate	Soy Acidophilus

Natural Chemo Protocols:

Vitamin B17 and Sour Sop leaves.

Anti-Oxidant Shots:
Anti-Oxidants help to destroy free radicals, which cause cancer in the body.

I call this "My vitamin Anti-oxidant shot" It is made up of one ounce of Mangosteen, one ounce of Noni, one ounce of Acai Berry, and one ounce of Gogi Berry. All 100% Juices.

IP 6 with Inositol:
This is a supplement I used to help boost my immune system.

For more information contact: A health food store nearest you.

Colonics:
Colonics could be done at a professional center.

Enemas:

An enema bag can be purchased at any pharmacy.
I will be honest with you, doing enemas was
unpleasant for me. I had to lay naked on my side to do
them. I had to put embarrassment out of my mind and
allow my caretaker to assist and teach me what to do.
These protocols were used to pull feces and toxins out
of my body.
When the body is healthy and working normally these
artificial means are not necessary, but when cancer is
present the body organs may not be at its optimum. I
did two enemas per day, for ten days, then I continued
once per week during the months of my recovery. I did
plain water enemas and coffee enemas.

To Prepare the Coffee:

Use 3 Table spoons of organic coffee to one quart of
water. Let this boil for about five minutes. Let it cool,
strain, and fill the enema bag when ready to use.

Fill the Enema bag with the liquid, either water or
coffee. Be sure to test flush it over the bathroom sink,
by allowing some liquid to flow out of the tubing
before closing the bag. This will release any air in the
tubing. Position the enema bag at the height of about
four feet from the ground. After lying down on the side
of the body, bring both knees up towards the chest.
Lubricate inside the rectum with a little Vaseline using

a gloved finger. Insert the erected end of the enema into the rectum until it is all the way inside. Lightly open the tube so that fluid begin to flow inside the rectum. Allow the water or coffee to go in slowly until the bag is empty. Lightly rub the stomach. If it becomes painful take a deep breath and short puffs till the pain passes. (Sometimes when the liquid meets gas it becomes painful). You will feel like you cannot hold it and you want to go to the bathroom, but, breathe through the feeling and hold the water in for as long as you can. I was only able to hold mine for about ten to fifteen minutes. As expected, I had to run to the toilet before passing out lots of debris. I was shocked that so much came out of me. I even observed mucous in my stool. As a reaction I experienced rumblings in my belly, chills and a cold feeling over my body in the beginning. I took a warm bath and covered with a warm blanket. Be sure to do your enema very close to the bathroom. Try not to do enemas pass the ten days of cleansing if your body will allow it. Be sure to have someone present with you. Remember to take an Acidophilus pill after the cleaning. This replaces the friendly bacteria in the system. This actually worked for me and I was relieved.

Hot and cold showers:

Hot and cold showers help to stimulate the immune system. I believe that God has made us so wonderful that our bodies can help heal itself. Our immune system should be kept as strong as possible to help us fight cancer cells. I showered with hot water for a few minutes, and then I switched to cold water for a few seconds. I repeated this process about four times, hot, then cold, hot then cold. Do this about four times and was careful to end with the cold water. Hot water opens the pores, and cold water closes them back. This protocol helps to stimulate the skin cells, improve circulation, and boosts the immune system.

Some delicious and helpful recipes:

Oat Burgers:
4 ½ cups water
4 ½ cups old-fashioned oats
1 diced onion
¼ cup yeast flakes
¾ cup walnuts or sunflower seeds
1/3 cup oil
½ cup Bragg's Liquid Aminos
1 tsp. garlic powder
¼ cup sesame seeds
Cook oats in boiling water and liquid aminos for five minutes. Mix remaining ingredients in a separate bowl. Add dry ingredients to cooked oats and mix well.

When cool enough to handle, form into patties, place on an oiled cookie sheet, and bake at 350 degrees for 30 to 45 minutes, turning halfway through cooking time, to brown on each side. May be frozen cooked or uncooked for future use.

Vegetarian Walnut Pate:

3 c. soaked walnuts
3 T. lemon juice
5-6 cloves garlic
3 t. flax oil
¼ c. fresh chopped parsley
¼ t. sea salt
3 T. fresh onion (chopped)
3 T. Bragg's Liquid Aminos or 1 T. sea salt

Process in food processor or blend in a blender. Do not over-process as pate should have some chunks in it.

Vegetarian -Nut Loaf:

Mix 2 Tbsp. oil
Add 1 ¼ cups soy or nut milk
2 Tbsp. flour or gluten-free flour
1 ¼ t. salt
Stir over heat until mixture boils. Then combine with:
2 c. chopped pecans, almonds or walnuts
¼ c. chopped onions
2 c. steamed brown rice, fluffy
1 c. finely chopped green pepper
2 Tbs. almond butter

2 c. seasoned breadcrumbs or gluten-free oats
Stir and mix well all together. Placed in a greased loaf
pan. Bake at 350 degrees F for 50-60 min. Turn out on
the platter. Serve with parsley or favorite gravy.

Fruit Smoothie recipe:

The base for the smoothie:
Almond, Cashews, Rice or Soy milk base. Make sure milk
is organic, and soy is not GMO.
Add frozen fresh fruit of different combinations.
Use Strawberries and raspberries as one choice
Or Blueberries and pineapple
Or Mango with pineapple and a little orange-note if using
these 3 fruits, put no milk at all!
Or ½ Avocado with nut or soya milk
Add 2 frozen bananas
1 C. milk of your choice
1 lemon freshly squeezed
Few dates to taste!
Ice to taste. Blend well. Serve.

Green Smoothie recipe:

(No fruit) This is a green smoothie with kale greens
and no banana or fruit.

1 c. kale or collard greens, packed (fresh)
½ medium avocado
2 T. chia seeds
½ c. lemon/ginger/or Echinacea drink
3 Brazil nuts
2 T. maple syrup
1 T. fresh lemon juice
Ice to taste. Blend well. Serve.

Raw Vegetable Plate:

Raw yam or sweet potato slices
Fresh Jicama-cut into French fry slices
Red bell pepper slices
Zucchini slices
Yellow squash slices
Place on bed of fresh arugula or spinach Serve with
Herb Cheese Dip or Creamy Dill Dressing

Herb Cheese Dip:

¾ C. almonds
¼ C. red onion stalk
1 T. fresh or dried dill
1 clove garlic
¼ C. pine nuts
2 T. fresh or dried parsley
1 T. nutritional yeast flakes
2 T. BL Aminos

Process in food processor until smooth.

Raw Vegetable Salad:

Shredded green cabbage
Shredded red cabbage
Shredded beets and shredded carrots
Top with Kalamata or ripe green olives, and chopped
green onions
Serve with Creamy Italian Salad Dressing
Very popular salad… serves well with short grain
brown rice and delicious black beans for a complete
meal.

<u>Creamy Italian Salad Dressing:</u>
2½ c. purified water
½ c. lemon juice
1tsp. garlic powder
1 tsp. Italian seasoning
¾ c. sesame
1 tsp. sea salt
2 tsp. onion powder
1 1/2 c. cashews or sunflower seeds
½ tsp. sweet basil
1 Tbsp. honey
Chill. Blend. Serve over your favorite salad.[24]

---

[24] All recipes taken from the following source:
Shorter, Rick and Gwen. Shorter's Health Manual Recipes for
Vegetarian Cooking and Nutrition Classes Washington: Homeward
Publishing (2017 4th Edition) Phone 1-800-823-0481
homewardpublishingministries@gmail.com
www.homewardpublishingministries.com

References:

Blahd, W. Reviewed this article (2016, December 21). What Is HER2-Positive Breast Cancer? WebMD Medical Reference, Retrieved from https://www.webmd.com/breast-cancer/qa/what-is-her2positive-breast-cancer

Cancer survivor. Quote found in paragraph two, sentence three. Retrieved from https://en.wikipedia.org/wiki/Cancer_survivor

Cancer-something you cannot be prepared for? (2017, August 5) Category: Medicine. Retrieved from https://mypassionmedicine.wordpress.com/category/medicine/

Cancer Survivor. Quote found in paragraph two, sentence two. Retrieved from https://en.wikipedia.org/wiki/Cancer_survivor

Cell food information adapted and Retrieved from http://www.naturesunique.net/CELL_FOOD.HTM

Comrie Millicent, Md.-Center for Women's Health - Brooklyn, NY.

Gaynor, Gloria. Lyrics. I Will Survive

Holland, K. (2016, January 13) What does a breast cancer lump feels like? Learn the symptoms. Medically reviewed by Christina Chun. (2017, October 11) Retrieved from https://www.healthline.com/health/what-does-breast-cancer-feel-like

Hawkins, Tramaine. Lyrics. What Should I Do?

Jolie. A. My Medical Choice, by Staff Reporter. (2013, May 14), paragraph 16. Retrieved from http://www.destinyconnect.com/2013/05/14/my-medical-choice-angelina-jolie-2013-05-14/

Leveillee, C. About Synervation. (A). Retrieved from http://www.synervationpt.com/about.html

Monod. A. Quotes. Swiss Clergyman (1800-1856). Retrieved from http://www.winwisdom.com/quotes/author/adolphe-monod.aspx

Macomber, Debbie - Quote

NCI Dictionary of Cancer Terms. Metastasis. Retrieved from www.cancer.gov/publications/dictionaries/cancer-terms/def/metastasis

Pathak, N. Reviewed this article (2018, January

30). Retrieved from
www.webmd.com/breast-cancer/when-breast-cancer-spreads

Pauley, J. (Adapted from the J.P. Story)

Ratini, M. Reviewed this article (2016, July 22).
What Does Cancer Remission Really Mean? -WebMD,
Retrieved from
https://www.webmd.com/cancer/remission-what-does-it-mean

Shorter, Rick and Gwen. Shorter's Health
Manual Recipes for Vegetarian Cooking and Nutrition
Classes Washington: Homeward Publishing (2017 4th
Edition) Phone 1-800-823-0481
homewardpublishingministries@gmail.com
www.homewardpublishingministries.com

Synergy Definition, *Business Dictionary.com*

Warburg, O.H. The Root Cause of Cancer,
Ganodermareview, Nobel Prize Winner. Retrieved
from
https://sites.google.com/site/ganodermareview/the-root-cause-of-cancer

What does cancer feel like? Pain: Obvious

Symptom That Cancer Can Cause. Retrieved from
https://www.newhealthadvisor.com/What-Does-
Cancer-Feel-Like.html

White, E.G. (1990) Desire of Ages. Silver
Springs: Review & Herald and Pacific Press, p. 203

White, E.G. Education, Ch. 21. Study of
Physiology, p. 96.1.

White E.G. Education Ch. 22. Temperance and
Dietetics, p. 205.4

About the Author

Ann Marie Fraser is a sought-after Health and Wealth Coach, who has addressed large and small audiences at hotels, churches, schools, and conventions around the country, and overseas.

She is a Certified Public Accountant, licensed in the State of New York. She holds a Bachelor's degree in accounting and a Master of Taxation from the Long Island University in Brooklyn, New York. For many years she has been helping churches and hundreds of ordinary people take good care of their taxes.

She has also built a career in Insurance and Financial Services and holds Life & Health licenses in several States. She enjoys presenting Financial and Health Seminars on a wide range of topics, including Business, Finance, Insurance, Estate & Retirement Planning, Taxation, Laws of Health, and Long-Term Care. She is a member of the National Association of Tax Professionals (NATP) and the National Notary Association (NNA).

Ann Marie's passion in life is to inspire women to use their God-given talents to build WEALTH and motivate them to practice a HEALTHY lifestyle while doing it. Through her 1on 1 coaching and group masterminds, she is helping dozens of women take their lives back by inspiring them to implement their Personal Financial Strategy.

As a motivator, her upbeat energy and attitude inspires her audience to reach their greatest potential. She is always excited to share common-sense financial, sales, marketing, and leadership experience with you.

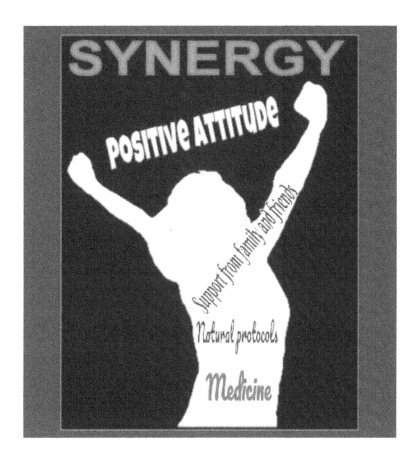

For book purchase, connect with us at:
Website: www.commonsensecancer.com
Email: info@annmariefraser.com
Fax: 718-789-0439
Phone: 646-645-0102

Made in the USA
Monee, IL
26 July 2021

74020959R00105